Date Due

BRODART, CO.   Cat. No. 23-233-003   Printed in U.S.A.

B. Heymer **Clinical and Diagnostic Pathology
of Graft-versus-Host Disease**

Springer

Berlin
Heidelberg
New York
Barcelona
Hong Kong
London
Milan
Paris
Tokyo

Berno Heymer

Clinical and Diagnostic Pathology of Graft-versus-Host Disease

With the Collaboration of
Donald Bunjes and Wilhelm Friedrich

With 55 Color Figures in 83 Separate Illustrations
and 21 Tables

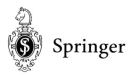

Springer

DEC 0 7 2002

Collaborators

PD Dr. Donald Bunjes
Abteilung Innere Medizin III, Universitätsklinikum Ulm
Robert-Koch-Straße 8, 89081 Ulm, Germany

Prof. Dr. Wilhelm Friedrich
Universitäts-Kinderklinik und Poliklinik
Prittwitzstraße 43, 89075 Ulm, Germany

ISBN 3-540-67719-4 Springer-Verlag Berlin Heidelberg New York

Library of Congress Cataloging-in-Publication Data
Heymer, Berno, 1936-. Clinical and diagnostic pathology of graft-versus-host disease (GvHD)/[Berno Heymer].
p.; cm. Includes bibliographical references and index.
ISBN3540677194 (alk. paper)
1. Graft versus host disease. I. Title. [DNLM: 1. Graft vs Host Disease - pathology. 2. Graft vs Host Disease - etiology. 3. Graft vs Host Disease - immunology. 4. Post-operative Complications. 5. Transplantation - adverse effects. WD 300 H618c 2002]
RD123.5.H49 2002   617.9'5-dc21   2001049884

Springer-Verlag Berlin Heidelberg New York
a member of BertelsmannSpringer Science+Business Media GmbH
http://www.springer.de

© Springer-Verlag Berlin Heidelberg 2002
Printed in Germany

The use of general descriptive names, registered names, trademarks, etc. in this publication does not imply, even in the absence of a specific statement, that such names are exempt from the relevant protective laws and regulations and therefore free for general use.
Product liability: The publishers cannot guarantee the accuracy of any information about dosage and application contained in this book. In every individual case the user must check such information by consulting the relevant literature.

Cover design: E. Kirchner, Heidelberg
Typesetting: Fotosatz-Service Köhler GmbH, Würzburg
Printing: Schneider Druck GmbH, Rothenburg ob der Tauber
Binding: J. Schäffer GmbH & Co. KG, Grünstadt

Printed on acid-free paper   SPIN 10753980   24/3130/op 5 4 3 2 1 0

To Annerose Heymer

Preface

A medical book need not be pretty, but it must be necessary and informative.

This monograph on the clinical and diagnostic pathology of graft-versus-host disease, providing detailed visual information on the histomorphological and immunohistological features of GvHD, is intended to close a gap in the otherwise comprehensive medical literature on GvHD.

B. Heymer

Acknowledgements

No one accumulates knowledge alone.
I owe thanks to:

Prof. G.R.F. Krüger, Houston, for introducing me
to the histomorphological analysis of GvHD

Prof. R. Arnold, Berlin, for many fruitful clinicopathological discussions

Prof. K.H. Müller-Hermelink, Würzburg, for
expert advice in difficult histological differential
diagnoses

Prof. W. Mohr, Ulm, for continuous support and
encouragement in moments of fatigue

Last, but by no means least, Mrs. R. Endres-Klein,
Ulm, without whom the preparation of this book
would have been impossible

In addition, I am grateful to the editorial staff at
Springer, Heidelberg.

B. Heymer

Contents

Abbreviations

AA	Aplastic anemia
ABC	Avidin-biotin complex
AEC	Aminoethylcarbazole
AIC	Autoimmune cholangitis
ALL	Acute lymphoblastic leukemia
AML	Acute myeloid leukemia
AUL	Acute undifferentiated leukemia
BCG	Bacillus Calmette-Guérin
BMSC	Bone marrow stem cell
BMT	Bone marrow transplantation
CB	Cord blood
CBSCT	Cord blood stem cell transplantation
CD	Cluster designation
CML	Chronic myeloid leukemia
CMV	Cytomegalovirus
CSA	Cyclosporine A
CTL	Cytotoxic T-lymphocyte
CY	Cyclophosphamide
DLI	Donor lymphocyte infusion
FA	Fanconi anemia
G-CSF	Granulocyte colony-stimulating factor
GIT	Gastrointestinal tract
GvHD	Graft-versus-host disease
GvHR	Graft-versus-host reaction
GvL	Graft-versus-leukemia
H&E	Hematoxilin and eosin
HCV	Hepatitis C virus
HLA	Human leukocyte antigen
HSC	Hematopoietic stem cell
HSCT	Hematopoietic stem cell transplantation
HSV	Herpes simplex virus
HvGR	Host-versus-graft reaction
IBMTR	International bone marrow transplant registry
ICAM	Intercellular adhesion molecule
IFN	Interferon
IHC	Immunohistochemistry

IL	Interleukin
ISH	In situ hybridization
MDS	Myelodysplastic syndrome
MFT	Materno-fetal transfusion
MHC	Major histocompatibility complex
MTX	Methotrexate
NK cell	Natural killer cell
PBC	Primary biliary cirrhosis
PBSC	Peripheral blood stem cell
PBSCT	Peripheral blood stem cell transplantation
PCR	Polymerase chain reaction
RAG	Recombination activating gene
RD	Reticular dysgenesis
SCID	Severe combined immunodeficiency
SOT	Solid organ transplantation
TA	Transfusion-associated
TBI	Total body irradiation
Th1, Th2	T-helper cell type 1 or type 2
TNF	Tumor necrosis factor
TUNEL	Terminal deoxynucleotidyl transferase (TdF)-mediated dUTP-biotin nick end labeling
VCAM	Vascular cell adhesion molecule
VOD	Venoocclusive disease
VZV	Varicella zoster virus
ZN	Ziehl-Neelsen

1 Introduction

1.1 What Is Graft-Versus-Host Disease?

Graft-versus-host disease (GvHD) is the mirror image of allograft rejection. In GvHD not the graft but the host is rejected. This rejection is mediated by alloreactive donor T-lymphocytes recognizing minor or major histocompatibility antigens on target tissues of the host. GvHD primarily affects skin, liver, and gastrointestinal tract (GIT), but it can also involve other organs and tissues. The mortality of severe forms of acute GvHD can be very high, ranging from 50% to 90% [139].

Most often GvHD occurs as a complication of allogeneic hematopoietic stem cell transplantation (HSCT), a life-saving measure and the treatment of choice for many patients with various severe malignant or nonmalignant diseases. During this procedure a certain number of allogeneic donor T-lymphocytes are cotransferred into the recipient in addition to hematopoietic stem cells (HSCs). These T-lymphocytes may then induce a most unusual immunopathological process. However, GvHD can also develop in a number of other settings such as materno-fetal transfusion, blood transfusion, solid organ transplantation, donor lymphocyte infusion and, allegedly, after autologous HSCT.

1.2 Has the Pathology of GvHD Changed in the Past Decades?

Within the past 20 years the number of allogeneic HSCTs has increased steadily [19, 42, 105, 322]. However, since 70% of potential transplant recipients do not have a suitable donor [8, 204], techniques have been developed that make possible the use of HSCs from alternative donors such as HLA (human leukocyte antigen)-nonidentical family members and HLA-identical or nonidentical unrelated volunteers [23, 233, 320]. The increased risk of GvHD encountered with such transplant modalities can be reduced by T-cell depletion of the graft [52, 233] or by intensified GvHD prophylaxis of patients [16, 75, 204]. On the one hand, these new preparative and prophylactic possibilities have permitted a significant expansion of the indications for allogeneic HSCT [19, 74, 248]. On the other hand, the increased use of unrelated or HLA-mismatched donors has caused GvHD to remain an important issue [19, 52, 70, 320].

Paradoxically, the improvements in HSC grafting and GvHD prophylaxis have not only reduced the incidence and severity of acute GvHD [16,75,245], but at the same time have rendered the histomorphological diagnosis of GvHD more difficult [66, 227, 352]. This is due to the fact that, in recent years, the number of histologically typical lesions has decreased and the number of atypical, low-grade, or masked lesions has increased [330,335]. In other words, nowadays the pathologist primarily gets to see what effective GvHD-prophylaxis or treatment have left over. Biopsies showing the histomorphological characteristics of full blown acute GvHD, recognizable at one glance, are the exception and not the rule. A histological diagnosis of GvHD today means a diagnosis in the presence of immunosuppressive GvHD-inhibiting drugs. Therefore, a reappraisal of GvHD histomorphology as it appears today is indicated.

1.3 Why Write a Synopsis of the Clinical and Diagnostic Pathology of GvHD?

There are a number of comprehensive books on organ transplantation [31, 183, 267] and bone marrow transplantation [18, 51, 74, 169, 323, 325] containing one or two chapters on the histomorphology of GvHD. In addition, there is a very informative monograph on the pathology of bone marrow transplantation with a detailed description of the histomorphology of acute and chronic GvHD [271]. Finally a comprehensive, excellent volume presenting all the various aspects of GvHD has been published [100]. Thus, without doubt, enough competent texts on the clinical as well as the pathological features of GvHD are available.

However, up to the present what still is lacking is a concise overview of the clinical and diagnostic pathology of GvHD with ample colored illustrations showing the various macroscopic and microscopic features of GvHD lesions. The primary objective of the present publication is therefore not simply to copy the already existing informative texts, but rather to provide an update of the histomorphology and immunohistology of GvHD. It will cover the whole spectrum of the histopathology of GvHD as it presents in the modern era of intensive GvHD – prophylaxis and therapy. Furthermore, this volume will focus attention on GvHD as a pathomorphological phenomenon which is not restricted to the HSCT setting but also occurs in a variety of other clinical situations. The etiology, pathogenesis, and clinical features of GvHD are dealt with only insofar as this is necessary for the understanding of the histopathology of GvHD.

Although animal experimental studies may be useful for the study of many aspects of GvHD, the present monograph is primarily based on studies in the human. There are several reasons for this restriction:

1. The histopathology of GvHD lesions in animal and human shows important differences.
2. The diagnostic potential of the histomorphological assessment of GvHD may depend on subtle histological features.
3. The emphasis of the present monograph is focused on the clinical and diagnostic pathology of GvHD in man as visible in tissue specimens available for routine pathology.

Thus, more precisely the prime objective of this book is twofold, namely, to present:

1. A concise well-illustrated overview of the clinical pathology of GvHD
2. An instructive, reliable guide to the histomorphological diagnosis of GvHD

The present volume has been written from the point of view of a pathologist who over the past 20 years has been asked almost daily by his clinical colleagues sending a biopsy: Is the histological finding compatible with GvHD? Whereas this question was relatively easy to answer in the past, in the last few years the answer has become more and more difficult and sometimes impossible. The reasons for these increasing diagnostic difficulties have already been mentioned. These facts thus raise questions such as:

- Is histology still a useful tool for the study of GvHD?
- What are the histomorphological correlates of clinically evident GvHD today?
- Are there histological parameters pathognomonic for GvHD?
- What are the clues to the histomorphological diagnosis of GvHD?
- How reliable is the histological diagnosis under the conditions of today?
- Do histomorphological parameters have prognostic relevance?
- Can immunohistological parameters assist in the recognition of GvHD?
- Are formalin-fixed paraffin-embedded tissues suitable for the immunohistological assessment of GvHD?
- Are there immunohistological features specific for GvHD?
- Do immunohistological markers permit an early diagnosis of GvHD?

In the following text an attempt is made to answer these questions.

2 Occurrence of GvHD

Allogeneic hematopoietic stem cell transplantation (HSCT), today, is the treatment of choice for life-threatening diseases such as aplastic anemia (AA), severe combined immunodeficiency (SCID), leukemia, and many other diseases [69]. The spectrum of indications for allogeneic HSCTs has steadily increased in recent years. At present approximately 20,000 allogeneic or autologous HSCTs are performed worldwide every year [70]. Thus, it is not surprising that GvHD most often occurs in the context of allogeneic HSCT. However, as is evident from Table 2.1, GvHD can also develop in other quite different clinical situations. Before this is outlined in more detail, it should be stressed that the manifestation of GvHD depends on a number of immunological as well as nonimmunological factors, such as:

1. The degree of histoincompatibility between donor and recipient [8, 23]
2. The type of conditioning regimen employed [151]
3. The number of allogeneic donor T-lymphocytes transferred [220]
4. The type of GvHD prophylaxis used [52, 75, 245]
5. The age of donor and recipient [159, 255]
6. The microbial flora or infection of the recipient [27, 255]

These and other factors strongly influence the incidence, onset, severity, course, and outcome of GvHD.

Table 2.1. Occurrence of GvHD

1. Bone marrow transplantation (BMT)
2. Peripheral blood stem cell transplantation (PBSCT)
3. Cord blood stem cell transplantation (CBSCT)
4. Materno-fetal transfusion (MFT)
5. Blood transfusion associated (TA)
6. Donor lymphocyte infusion (DLI)
7. Solid organ transplantation (SOT)

2.1 GvHD After Allogeneic Bone Marrow Transplantation

Allogeneic bone marrow grafts contain a variable number of mature T-lymphocytes in addition to a relatively heterogenous population of HSCs [344]. These T-cells can induce GvHD in the recipient. After HLA-identical sibling bone marrow transplantation (BMT) the incidence of acute GvHD is 35%–50% and the incidence of chronic GvHD 40%–50% of long-term survivors [19,73]. When HLA-nonidentical BMT is performed the probability of severe acute GvHD increases to 50%–60% [23]. However, if such patients are given a combined GvHD prophylaxis of methotrexate (MTX) and cyclosporine A (CSA) a reduced rate and a delayed onset of GvHD is observed [8]. GvHD prophylaxis with CSA/MTX usually prevents severe acute GvHD after HLA-identical sibling transplantation, but not always after HLA-identical unrelated donor transplantation [19].

When patients receive HLA-identical sibling transplants depleted of T-cells the incidence of acute GvHD is 4% instead of 35% and that of chronic GvHD 3% instead of 36% [129]. This indicates that T-lymphocytes play an important role in the pathogenesis of GvHD.

The significance of the "age" factor in HLA-identical BMT is illustrated by an incidence of acute GvHD of 25% or less in patients under 30 years and of approximately 80% in patients over 50 years of age [305]. Data in patients with AA receiving transplants from HLA-identical sibling donors are similar: While the risk of acute GvHD is 15%–20% in children, it reaches 40%–45% in adults over 40 years of age [159]. Finally, it is important to point out that adults also have a higher incidence and severity of chronic GvHD than children [23,159].

The incidence and mortality of acute GvHD can be significantly reduced by treatment of bone marrow transplant recipients with certain antibiotics [27] and/or by treatment of patients in a protective environment [255]. This indicates that microbes, in particular the intestinal anaerobic bacterial flora, play a role in the clinical manifestation of acute GvHD after allogeneic BMT.

2.2 GvHD After Allogeneic Peripheral Blood Stem Cell Transplantation

Whereas bone marrow was for many years the sole source of HSCs, hematopoietic progenitor cells circulating in the peripheral blood of patients have been increasingly used for transplantation in recent years [47, 204]. These CD34+ peripheral blood stem cells (PBSCs), in contrast to bone marrow stem cells (BMSCs), represent a relatively uniform cell population [344]. By treatment of donors with granulocyte colony-stimulating factor (G-CSF) PBSCs can be mobilized and obtained in relatively large numbers [62]. The engraftment of such PBSCs in the tissues of recipients, as compared to BMSCs, is considerably accelerated [47]. This more rapid and sustained engraftment has the advantage of a faster granulocyte, platelet, and immunological recovery [19, 47, 61, 282].

Allogeneic CD34$^+$ PBSCs do not directly cause GvHD [233]. However, unmanipulated PBSC preparations contain ten to a hundred times more T-lymphocytes than bone marrow grafts [29, 30, 304]. This should normally increase the risk of developing GvHD. Surprisingly, clinical experience with allogeneic PBSCT has failed to show a higher incidence or severity of acute GvHD in most studies [29, 47, 61, 250]. There is, however, some evidence suggesting that patients experience chronic GvHD more frequently (37% – 72%) after the transplantation of PBSCs than after the transplantation of BMSCs (30% – 50%; [30, 61, 176, 282, 304]) . However, this question has not yet been answered definitely [250].

2.3 Alternative Donors

Until recently the majority of allogeneic BMTs or PBSCTs were performed from HLA-identical siblings. However, only 30% of patients have a suitable donor [204]. Therefore, alternative donors (HLA-nonidentical family members, unrelated volunteers) are used for transplantation with increasing frequency [47, 248]. If positive selection of G-CSF mobilized peripheral blood CD34$^+$ progenitors are employed for the depletion of T-lymphocytes [233], the transplantation of megadoses of HLA-haploidentical stem cells is possible in pediatric and adult patients without inducing clinically significant GvHD [131]. In non T-cell-depleted transplants the increasing use of alternative donors has, however, turned GvHD into a major clinical problem.

2.4 Umbilical Cord Blood

Another alternative to BMT is the use of umbilical cord blood (CB) as a source for CD34$^+$ hematopoietic stem/progenitor cells [122]. Such cells circulate in fetal blood and after birth can be easily isolated from the placenta through the umbilical cord [62]. The first successful transplantation of CB stem cells in man was reported in 1989 [121]. Subsequently it was found that such cells mediate prompt and sustained multilineage engraftment [233, 340] and that the risk of severe GvHD is relatively low [50, 62, 65, 263]. This even holds true for the HLA-mismatched situation [192, 324].

There are several possible reasons for the low incidence and severity of acute GvHD after CB stem cell transplantation (CBSCT). CB contains a lower number of alloreactive T-cell precursors than peripheral blood of adults [340]. Moreover, it has been observed that immunotolerance to maternal and paternal antigens persists in the newborn for about 6 months after birth

[132]. During this time CB lymphocytes are nonresponsive to alloantigens from the mother or father [340]. Also, there is evidence that CB cells are immunologically immature [122, 132]. This is indicated by their reduced capacity for cytokine production [58, 185]. Thus, CB lymphocytes produce less interleukin-2 (IL-2), IL-4, interferon-γ (IFNγ) and tumor necrosis factor-α (TNFα) than peripheral blood lymphocytes of adults [50].

The estimated incidence of acute GvHD in recipients of CB from HLA-identical related donors is only 9% and in recipients of CB from HLA-mismatched related donors 37% – 50% [122, 324]. After unrelated CB transplantation no GvHD is observed in 31%, mild GvHD in 25%, moderate GvHD in 22% and severe GvHD in 22% [263, 264]. The incidence and severity of acute GvHD after CB transplantation corresponds to the degree of HLA incompatibility between donor and recipient. Chronic GvHD, occurring in 23% – 25% of patients, correlates with prior acute GvHD but not with HLA disparity [263, 264].

The main disadvantage of CB transplantation is its limitation to younger patients, because of the low dose of HSCs available. Therefore, most adults and larger children are not suitable for CBSCT [160].

2.5 GvHD After Materno-fetal Transfusion

During pregnancy maternal blood cells occasionally cross the placental barrier and reach the fetal circulation [42]. If the fetus is immunocompetent these cells will be eliminated rapidly [232]. However, if the fetus suffers from SCID, maternal cells, e.g., T-lymphocytes, cannot be destroyed, but may persist in the fetus and induce GvHD [14, 42, 113]. In contrast to most forms of GvHD which represent an iatrogenic complication, GvHD following intrauterine materno-fetal transfusion (MFT) develops spontaneously.

The presence of maternal cells in fetal tissues can be detected by HLA typing [103] or by Y-chromosome-specific polymerase chain reaction (PCR) amplification analysis [13]. While intrauterine MFT and engraftment of maternal T-cells in fetuses with SCID occurs frequently (in about 50% of cases; [105, 280]), the development of clinically manifest GvHD in such fetuses is rare [6, 42, 103, 113, 143, 280, 301].

The clinical symptoms of GvHD following MFT in infants with SCID in most instances are mild and require no or only transient steroid treatment [42, 301]. However, marked GvHD with erythema, diarrhea, and hepatitis also has been observed in this situation [62].

Finally, it has been suggested that intrauterine or postnatal cryptic GvHD might be an important pathogenetic mechanism responsible for a variety of diseases in infancy and childhood [281]. Unfortunately, this possibility has not yet been studied in detail.

2.6 GvHD After Blood Transfusion

Transfusion-associated (TA) GvHD is a distinct disease entity [10, 246, 299]. It may occur after transfusion of nonirradiated blood or blood products in particular situations [134, 161, 252]. Most often TA-GvHD is observed in individuals with primary or secondary immunodeficiency [10, 41, 232, 237]. However, occasionally it may also develop in premature infants [135, 237] and even in immunocompetent healthy individuals [10, 124, 262, 331]. The occurrence of TA-GvHD in the latter is explained by a "one-way HLA match" between donor and recipient [10, 124]. Remarkably, the clinical course and outcome of TA-GvHD in immunocompetent individuals is not different from that in immunocompromised hosts.

TA-GvHD is induced by viable allogeneic T-cells present in blood or blood products used for transfusion. It is characterized by a rapid onset (8–10 days after transfusion), severe disease manifestations with fever, pancytopenia, multiorgan dysfunction, resistance to treatment, and a rapidly fatal course within 3–4 weeks in about 90% of patients [10, 237, 301]. Involvement of the bone marrow is a characteristic feature of TA-GvHD [246]. Lesions in skin, liver, and GIT are comparable to those found in acute GvHD induced by allogeneic BMT or PBSCT [12, 13, 301]. This statement is important since patients with TA-GvHD usually do not receive chemoradiation conditioning. Therefore, the histomorphology of their lesions cannot be ascribed to the effects of drugs and/or radiation.

The unequivocal diagnosis of TA-GvHD requires demonstration of donor lymphocytes in affected organs or lesions [135]. This can be accomplished by HLA typing [46, 232, 246] or, if donor and recipient are sex-mismatched, by in situ hybridization (ISH) of lesional biopsies with a Y-chromosome-specific probe [316]. It is important to note that lack of blood chimerism does not exclude TA-GvHD [135].

2.7 GvHD After Donor Lymphocyte Infusion

Donor T-cells present in the hematopoietic stem cell graft are not only responsible for inducing GvHD, they are also capable of exerting a powerful antileukemic activity which has been termed the graft-versus-leukemia (GvL) effect [40]. This GvL effect can be utilized to treat leukemic relapses after allogeneic HSCT [138, 181, 182]. The infusion of lymphocytes of the original stem cell donor (DLI) can induce complete remissions and is associated with an incidence of acute and chronic GvHD of approximately 50% if the donor is an HLA-identical sibling. The GvHD after allogeneic DLI is similar to TA-GvHD because the bone marrow in relapsed patients is a target organ for GvHD.

2.8 GvHD After Solid Organ Transplantation

The main problem of allogeneic organ transplantation is acute or chronic host versus graft reaction (HvGR), that is, allograft rejection. However, solid organ transplantation (SOT) can be complicated by a number of other problems such as infection, ischemia and, rarely, acute GvHD. In this instance, GvHD is induced by T-cells present in the organ transplant. This has been observed after transplantation of various organs, in particular following liver allografts [20, 44, 166, 230, 257].

The clinical manifestations of the disease are similar to those after allogeneic BMT or PBSCT. However, patients with acute GvHD following liver transplantation show two peculiarities: (1) The liver itself is not affected by GvHD since the alloreactive T-lymphocytes and the liver are derived from the same donor; and (2) pancytopenia is a prominent feature of this type of GvHD because the bone marrow of the recipient is a target for alloreactive donor T-lymphocytes [59].

The diagnosis of organ transplant-mediated GvHD is established by documenting donor chimerism through HLA-typing of the recipient [59, 226] or, in the sex-mismatched setting, by Y-chromosome-specific ISH [20].

It has been speculated that the risk of developing GvHD in this clinical context depends on the amount of viable lymphatic tissue present in the organ allograft: Small bowel → lung → liver → kidney → heart [166].

If one takes into account the rarity of proven SOT-GvHD it is hard to say whether such a risk scale is valid or not. However, some authors assume that GvHD in the setting discussed might be considerably underdiagnosed [166, 226]. This is compatible with the observation that microchimerism of $CD34^+$ cells in long-term liver allograft recipients is frequent [230].

2.9 GvHD After Autologous Bone Marrow or Peripheral Blood Stem Cell Transplantation?

According to Billingham [35] GvHD can develop only if there is a genetic difference between donor and host. This would imply that GvHD cannot manifest itself when histocompatibility barriers are absent. However, after autologous or syngeneic BMT or PBSCT about 8% – 10% of patients develop a skin rash that clinically [140], histomorphologically [33, 92], and immunohistochemically [92, 127] is indistinguishable from true GvHD [153]. Therefore, this phenomenon has been termed "autologous GvHD" [175]. Other designations are: auto-GvHD [53]; autoimmune GvHD [269]; pseudo-GvHD [269]; autoaggression GvHD-like syndrome [214]; acute GvHD-like syndrome [214]; GvHD-like cutaneous syndrome [33].

In addition, comparable skin lesions have been observed in 70%–80% of patients after recombinant IL-2 therapy [209] and following CSA withdrawal after autologous BMT [33, 53, 175].

"Autologous GvHD" shows a number of peculiarities [140, 175, 214, 286]: (1) It affects the skin only; other organs are not involved; (2) the skin rash has a transient, self-limiting character, resolving within 1–3 weeks either spontaneously or after a short course of steroid treatment; and (3) the rash typically manifests around the time of stem cell engraftment.

Many authors believe that "autologous GvHD," because of the clinical, histological, and immunohistochemical similarity with true GvHD, is in fact a variant of the latter. However, recipients of autologous or syngeneic HSCT, who have been irradiated and treated with CSA resulting in damage of the thymus, may lose self-tolerance and develop autoimmune reactivity [269]. Consequently, for the phenomenon discussed here, Sale [269] recommends the term "autoimmune GvHD" or "pseudo-GvHD" in order to distinguish it from true alloimmune GvHD. There are good reasons to follow this suggestion:

1. The similarity of the histological picture of alloimmune GvHD and "autoimmune GvHD" by no means implies that they are the same type of reaction. Histomorphological analogy does not prove etiopathogenetic identity [141].
2. Not every disease has a specific histological substrate. The organism possesses only a limited spectrum of histomorphologically distinct reactions. Therefore, the histological picture of many acute inflammatory reactions is relatively stereotyped [141].
3. Whereas true GvHD most characteristically is an alloimmune reaction, the phenomenon discussed here, mimicking GvHD, obviously is an autoimmune reaction [53].

If these arguments are taken into account, then the clinical, histological and immunohistochemical similarity of skin lesions developing after autologous or allogeneic HSCT does not prove the existence of an "autologous GvHD."

3 Pathogenesis of GvHD

The essential requirements for the induction of GvHD have been known since Billingham [35], in 1966, defined what is necessary:

"1. The graft must contain immunologically competent cells.
 2. The host must possess important transplantation isoantigens that are lacking in the graft donor, so that the host appears foreign to it and is therefore capable of stimulating it antigenically.
 3. The host itself must be incapable of mounting an effective immunological reaction against the graft, at least for sufficient time for the latter to manifest its immunological capabilities – i.e., the graft must have some security of tenure."

These statements, without doubt, still hold true today. Histoincompatibility is the most important factor in the pathogenesis of GvHD. The incidence, onset, and severity of GvHD correlates directly with the degree of HLA disparity between donor and recipient [8, 174]. However, as will be seen in the following, other factors are also involved.

Alloreactive T-lymphocytes play a central role in the pathogenesis of GvHD [11, 19, 74]. Within the past decade it has been found that cytokines are also involved [96, 98]. This is not surprising since cytokines participate in the development of practically all acute inflammatory processes [164]. In any event, it is true at present that some authors consider GvHD exclusively a manifestation of T-lymphocyte cytotoxicity whereas others regard such lesions primarily a consequence of cytokine-mediated tissue damage. The consensus appears to be that both mechanisms are involved in the pathogenesis of GvHD.

These few hints already indicate that GvHD is a complex, multifactorial process and that some aspects of its pathogenesis are still unknown. Since knowledge of the underlying pathogenetic pathways facilitates the understanding of the histomorphology of GvHD, they will be described briefly.

3.1 Activity of Allogeneic T-Lymphocytes

There is general agreement that alloreactive T-lymphocytes ultimately mediate the induction of GvHD. This has been shown locally within GvHD lesions, by analysis of peripheral blood of patients, by use of T-cell reactive immunosuppressive drugs, and, finally, by T-cell depletion of grafts used for allogeneic HSCT.

There are a number of studies which describe the phenotype and function of donor T-lymphocytes infiltrating GvHD lesions [9, 32, 171, 316]. These investigations provide evidence that both $CD8^+$ and $CD4^+$ T-cells are involved in the pathogenesis of GvHD. Donor T-lymphocytes present within lesions are host-reactive and possess either cytotoxic activity or release proinflammatory cytokines [118, 325].

Other studies indicate that the peripheral blood of patients with GvHD contains host-specific cytotoxic as well as cytokine-producing T-lymphocytes [93, 229, 231, 317, 318], which belong to both T-cell subtypes $CD8^+$ and $CD4^+$ [297]. However, monitoring of host-reactive T-lymphocytes in the peripheral blood of patients might not adequately reflect the local, intralesional pathophysiology [81, 171].

There is abundant evidence that T-cell-inhibiting agents such as cyclosporin A (CSA), frequently employed in combination with MTX, are effective in GvHD prophylaxis [74, 75, 220, 245]. CSA blocks T-cell activation [303] or, more specifically, blocks the release of interleukin-2 (IL-2) and other cytokines from activated T-lymphocytes [220]. However, while CSA/MTX usually prevents severe acute GvHD after HLA-identical sibling transplantation, this is not always the case after HLA-identical unrelated donor transplantation [19].

When HLA-identical or nonidentical HSCT is performed using transplants depleted of T-cells, no clinically relevant GvHD is observed [113]. When T-lymphocytes are eliminated by monoclonal antibodies from the transplants as well as the recipients, the incidence of acute GvHD is 7% as compared to 38% and of chronic GvHD 18% as compared to 45% in patients undergoing conventional nondepleted allogeneic HSCT [129, 130]. Consequently, T-cell depletion is a very effective measure for preventing GvHD [109, 114].

3.2 Activity of Cytokines

Cytokines are a group of biologically highly active polypeptides and glycoproteins that are produced by many different cell types and that trigger numerous cellular activities [64, 97, 190, 343]. They are thereby important mediators of immunity and inflammation [1]. There also is good evidence that cytokines are involved in the pathogenesis of acute GvHD [96, 101, 147,

333]. As a matter of fact, some investigators consider severe acute GvHD a paradigm of a "cytokine storm" [98, 102].

Cytokines active in acute GvHD can be derived from both donor and host tissues, from T-lymphocytes as well as from other cells [110]. Alloreactive T-lymphocytes of the donor can produce cytokines such as IFNγ and IL-2. Macrophages of the donor or the host may release cytokines such as TNFα and IL-1 [1]. So what is the evidence that cytokines do in fact play a role in the pathogenesis of GvHD?

Numerous studies have shown that the serum of patients with acute GvHD contains elevated levels of various cytokines such as TNFα, IFNγ, IL-1, IL-2, IL-6 [139, 150, 151, 152, 228, 259, 312]. However, the titer of most of these cytokines is not only increased during acute GvHD but also after conditioning with total body irradiation (TBI) and cyclophosphamide (CY) or in the course of microbial infections [150, 228, 259]. This indicates that their release is not GvHD-specific and that the determination of cytokine serum levels cannot be used for monitoring acute GvHD.

In contrast, elevated titers of soluble IL-2 receptor (sIL-2R) appear to correlate with the severity of the disease and therefore could be a reliable indicator of acute GvHD [125, 179]. This might also hold true for the level of soluble TNF-receptor [54], of IL-5 [163], and of IL-18 [116].

Another piece of evidence for the significance of cytokines in the pathogenesis of acute GvHD is provided by observations on the efficacy of cytokine blockade. The occurrence of acute GvHD can be significantly reduced, or at least the onset of acute GvHD postponed, by the prophylactic application of monoclonal anti-TNFα antibodies to patients undergoing HLA-identical sibling BMT [139, 151, 152]. Since CSA is known to inhibit production of cytokines by lymphocytes, the efficacy of CSA in GvHD prophylaxis points in the same direction [96, 120]. Plenty of evidence thus exists that the blockade of cytokines can delay the onset and reduce the severity of acute GvHD [146, 147].

As mentioned before, CD4$^+$ as well as CD8$^+$ T-cells are involved in the pathogenesis of GvHD. Both T-cell subsets can differentiate into type 1 and type 2 T-helper cells (Th1, Th2). Th1-cytokines such as IFNγ and IL-2 obviously participate in the development of acute GvHD [98, 110]. Because Th2-cytokines such as IL-4 or IL-10 can inhibit the production of proinflammatory Th1-cytokines, a Th1-Th2 shift might interrupt the cytokine cascade and thus prevent the manifestation of acute GvHD [98, 147]. In addition, this shift might possibly mediate the development of tolerance [97].

3.3 Combined Activity of Allogeneic T-Lymphocytes and Cytokines

From the data presented, it is evident that both T-lymphocytes and cytokines play an important role in the pathogenesis of acute GvHD [74, 98, 99, 100, 101, 102]. While alloreactive T-lymphocytes (CD4[+] and CD8[+]) obviously dominate in the inductive phase, cytokines may be prevalent in the effector phase of the pathogenesis of acute GvHD [110, 269]. However, there is evidence that cytokines, released by pretransplant conditioning, are involved also in the induction, and alloreactive cytotoxic T-lymphocytes also are involved in the manifestation of acute GvHD [98, 269]. Furthermore, it has been observed that natural killer (NK) cells and macrophages may contribute to the development of GvHD lesions [110, 155, 177, 254, 308]. Thus, the pathogenesis of acute GvHD, as far as known today, is more complex than originally thought. The observation that interruption of the development of acute GvHD in a more advanced stage requires blockade of T-cells as well as of cytokines in fact proves that both are involved [152].

The data reported indicate that acute GvHD is a multifactorial process with participation of immunologically specific as well as nonspecific mechanisms, of donor as well as host cells, of T-lymphocytes and accessory cells, and of biochemical mediators such as the cytokines [69, 70, 99, 100, 110, 147, 333]. A strongly simplified schematic representation of the pathogenesis of acute GvHD is shown in Fig. 3.1.

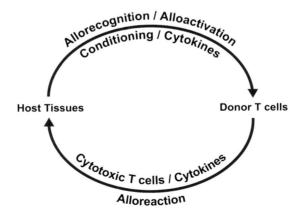

Fig. 3.1. Schematic representation of the pathogenesis of acute GvHD

As can be seen, during the inductive phase allogeneic donor T-cells recognize foreign major or minor histocompatibility antigens of host tissues. This leads to alloactivation and, after several intermediate stages, to formation of cytotoxic as well as cytokine-releasing T-cells. During the effector phase these alloreactive T-cells and cytokines attack target organs of the host such as skin, liver, and GIT causing GvHD (Fig. 3.1).

The interaction of allogeneic donor T-cells and host tissues can be influenced by many different factors. Indeed, the inductive phase can be triggered by cytokines released by the pretransplant conditioning of patients [102]. Similarly, the effector phase can be amplified by cytokines released from accessory cells such as macrophages [155, 177]. Although the schematic representation depicted in Fig. 3.1 no doubt oversimplifies the pathogenesis of acute GvHD, it does indicate the continuous interaction between donor and host. This may lead either to immunotolerance and stable chimerism or to GvHD [97].

3.4 Significance of Cofactors

Besides the special role played by histoincompatibility, a number of other factors may influence the incidence, onset, severity, and clinical course of GvHD. Such cofactors (risk factors) include the clinical context of the GvHD manifestation (see pp. 5–11), the age of patients, the underlying disease, the conditioning regimen, the microbial flora and infections of patients, the type of stem cell graft, the type of GvHD prophylaxis used, and others. The exact mode of action of most of these factors is still unknown. One possibility is that that some of the cofactors enhance alloreactivity by increasing major histocompatibility complex (MHC) antigen expression on GvHD target cells [96, 229]. Certainly, if one takes into account the complex pathogenesis of acute GvHD (see Fig. 3.1) there are definitely many more potential points of attack for cofactors that exacerbate GvHD.

3.4.1 Clinical Context

As previously described in detail, GvHD can occur in quite different clinical situations, e.g., after allogeneic BMT or PBSCT, after blood transfusion, or after MFT. Developing under these different conditions, GvHD varies considerably with respect to incidence, severity, and spectrum of target organs. Further, the manifestation of GvHD is influenced by the fact that some patients receive GvHD prophylaxis and some do not. A number of drugs or methods used for prophylaxis are listed in Table 3.1. Whereas the incidence of acute GvHD after HSCT may be 20%–30% with state of the art prophylaxis, it is 90%–100% if no prophylaxis is given [69, 70]. However, some of

Table 3.1. GvHD prophylaxis and treatment (modified from Deeg [70])

In vivo
  Methotrexate
  Azathioprine
  Cyclosporine
  Glucocorticoids
  Antithymocyte globulin
  Thalidomide
  Mycophenolate mofetil
  Rapamycin
  Cytokine antagonists
In vitro
  T-cell depletion by:
  Soybean lectin-agglutination
  Elutriation
  Column fractionation
  E-rosetting
  Monoclonal antibodies
  Immunotoxins

the substances listed in Table 3.1 (e.g., CSA, MTX) not only reduce the incidence and severity of acute GvHD, but also may induce toxic tissue changes mimicking acute GvHD. This must be kept in mind when analyzing lesions occurring in patients after GvHD prophylaxis.

3.4.2 Age of Patients

Incidence, onset, and severity of GvHD are significantly influenced by the age of patients [74, 100, 174]. Acute as well as chronic GvHD after HLA-identical BMT is much rarer in children, for example, than in adults [42]. This also holds true for haploidentical BMT [8].

3.4.3 Underlying Disease

Incidence, onset, and severity of GvHD also are affected by the underlying disease of patients [74, 100, 105]. In view of the fundamental differences that exist between diseases such as leukemia, AA, SCID, and other indications for HSCT, it is not surprising that there are differences in the development of GvHD. Before this issue is discussed in detail, one should remember that other factors known to influence GvHD manifestation such as age, pretransplant conditioning, and posttransplant prophylaxis may be inseparably connected with the underlying disease [218].

3.4.4 Pretransplant Conditioning

Prior to HSCT, patients suffering from malignant diseases such as leukemia are conditioned with irradiation and/or cytoreductive chemotherapy. This preparative regimen has a triple purpose:

1. To eradicate the underlying malignancy
2. To suppress immunological activity mediating allograft rejection and
3. To provide space in bone marrow for homing of donor stem cells

Such pretransplant conditioning (Table 3.2) can lead to tissue damage and release of cytokines such as TNFα, IL-1 or IL-6 [70]. These cytokines may activate donor T-cells or induce enhanced antigen presentation to donor T-cells [147]. The low incidence and mild, self-limited course of acute GvHD in infants with SCID after HLA-identical HSCT is due possibly to the lack of requirement for a pretransplant preparative regimen [42, 105]. This indicates that the conditioning-related cytokine release triggers an increased incidence and severity and an accelerated onset of acute GvHD [70, 96, 98, 110, 325, 333].

Nevertheless, as is evident from the occurrence of TA-GvHD in immunodeficient or immunocompetent adults, pretransplant conditioning is not a conditio sine qua non for the induction of GvHD [124]. This assertion is further supported by the development of GvHD in infants with SCID after allogeneic HSCT without pretransplant conditioning [161].

3.4.5 Microbial Flora and Infection

The incidence, onset, and severity of acute GvHD are significantly influenced by the intestinal flora and enteral infections of patients [27, 49, 174]. In particular endotoxin, a Gram-negative bacterial component of the normal bowel

Table 3.2. Pretransplant conditioning regimens

1. Total body irradiation (TBI)
2. Cytoablative chemotherapy (many different substances)
3. Combination of both regimens (used in most patients)

flora, is thought to play a role in the pathogenesis of acute GvHD [146]. Decontamination of patients with antibiotics targeted to intestinal anaerobic bacteria was shown to considerably reduce the severity of acute GvHD, supporting the hypothesis that such germs can be involved pathogenetically [27]. Viral infections such as cytomegalovirus (CMV) may also trigger the manifestation of GvHD [174].

3.4.6 Other Cofactors

There are still other risk factors for GvHD. For instance, the sex of patients plays a role sometimes. The incidence of GvHD is significantly higher in male patients given bone marrow from female donors than in male patients receiving sex-matched BMT [42]. The reason for this difference is the expression of male-specific minor histocompatibility antigens in male recipients (Y-antigen). Similarly, sensitization to host minor-histocompatibility antigens by multiple transfusions or multiple pregnancies may account for the higher rate of GvHD associated with the use of donors having a transfusion history or one of multiple pregnancies. The list of such pathogenetically important cofactors could be extended considerably.

Altogether, the multiplicity of factors involved make the pathogenesis of GvHD a very complex issue. However, the conditioning regimen employed, the type of GvHD-prophylaxis used, and the degree of immunodeficiency of the patient are of particular importance for the histomorphological appearance of GvHD lesions.

3.5 GvHD as an Inflammation Under the Conditions of Immunosuppression

Inflammatory lesions are the result of a highly complex interaction between the causative agent and the host. Their histological pattern reflects the properties of the causative agent as well as the properties of the host [141]. Therefore, infectious lesions induced in the immunocompromised ("defenseless") host are histomorphologically completely different from those in immunocompetent individuals. This holds true for lesions caused by pathogenic as well as by opportunistic germs [106, 212, 221, 270].

Just two examples for the atypical histomorphology of infectious lesions under the conditions of immunodeficiency: (1) While BCG (Bacillus Calmette-Guérin) vaccination of infants with SCID frequently causes BCG histiocytosis (Fig. 3.2), these microorganisms in the same patients, after allogeneic BMT and immunological reconstitution, induce epithelioid cell granulomata (Fig. 3.3). In other words, BCG histiocytosis after immunolog-

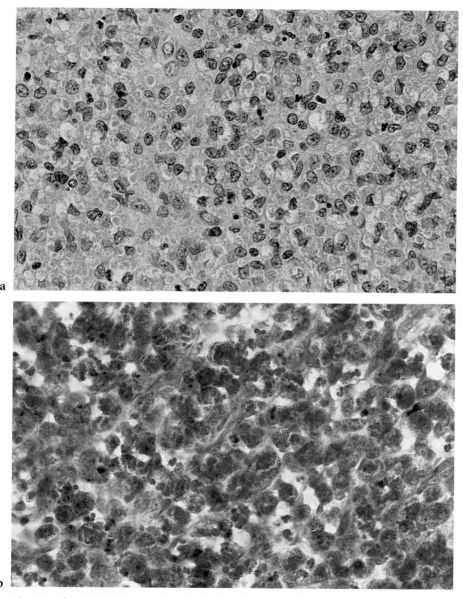

Fig. 3.2 a, b. BCG histiocytosis of skin in a 7-month-old male infant with SCID subsequent to BCG vaccination. **a** H & E staining: tissue infiltration by histiocytes only, no lymphocytes, no other inflammatory cells present. **b** Ziehl-Neelsen staining: abundant acid fast bacilli identifiable within histiocytes. **a, b** × 420

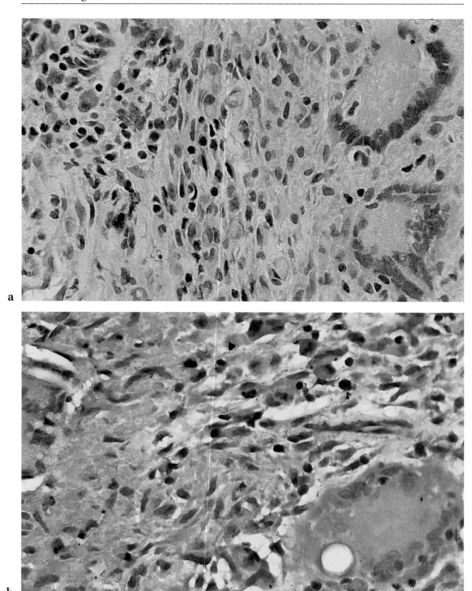

Fig. 3.3a, b. BCG granulomatosis of lymph node in a $7^{1}/_{2}$-month-old female infant with SCID subsequent to BCG vaccination. Biopsy $4^{1}/_{2}$ months after HLA-identical allogeneic BMT and immunological reconstitution. **a** H&E staining: granulomatous inflammation with lymphocytes and multinucleated giant cells. **b** Ziehl-Neelsen staining: no acid fast bacilli detectable in tissue. **a, b** ×420

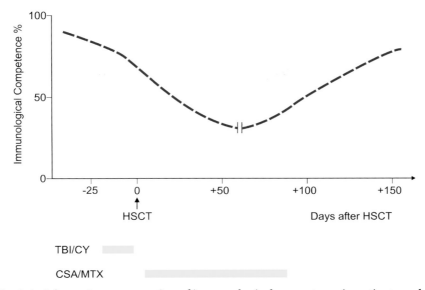

Fig. 3.4. Schematic representation of immunological competence in patients undergoing allogeneic HSCT. A transient state of strong immunosuppression is needed to allow take of allograft and inhibit allograft rejection. TBI, total body irradiation; CY, cyclophosphamide; CSA, cyclosporine A; MTX, methotrexate

ical reconstitution is transformed into BCG granulomatosis demonstrating rapid and efficient elimination of the pathogen. (2) Whereas pyogenic cocci in the immunocompetent individual elicit focal pyogenic inflammation (abscesses), the same germs induce diffuse areactive tissue necrosis in the immunocompromised host. The integrity of the immune system of patients is thus seen to have direct influence on the histomorphology of lesions.

Similarly, acute GvHD after HSCT represents an inflammation in the immunocompromised host. In fact, a transient state of maximal immunosuppression is a necessary prerequisite for the engraftment of allogeneic HSCs (Fig. 3.4). In this vulnerable period, in the first 3–5 months after HSCT, infections are very common. From the point of view of the histopathologist it is important to point out that acute GvHD, mediated by alloreactive donor T-cells, manifests in tissues of a host who is profoundly immuno- and myelosuppressed [68, 142, 346]. This means that the tissue will be insufficiently supplied with blood-derived cellular components. Therefore the delicate interaction of immunity, inflammation, and repair [38, 164] will not function properly. In other words, immunosuppression inhibits the inflammatory response [64]. The histomorphology of acute GvHD is therefore characterized by a discrepancy between the severity of tissue damage and the paucity of inflammatory infiltrate [98]. This disparity is not surprising but to be expected.

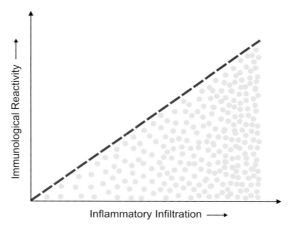

Fig. 3.5. Schematic representation of the relationship between immunological reactivity of the host and inflammatory infiltration of tissue

As a matter of fact, GvHD is an inflammatory reaction occurring in an organism that lacks many of the components of inflammation [141]. At the histomorphological level the situation is even more complex since GvHD represents an alloimmune reaction in a pathological, that is, a preconditioned and immunosuppressed microenvironment [76, 97, 291, 293]. A normal inflammatory reaction cannot develop in such tissues. Acute GvHD usually occurs around the onset of hematopoietic regeneration (Fig. 3.4). At this time alloreactive donor T-lymphocytes infiltrate the GvHD target tissues. However, with the exception of monocytes/macrophages, few accessory cells can be recruited from the host, and early-phase GvHD lesions frequently show a very sparse inflammatory infiltrate. This means that the field of inflammation in the GvHD target area is more or less "empty," histomorphologically elusive, and non-diagnostic.

The relationship between the immune state of the host and the inflammatory tissue reaction is depicted schematically in Fig. 3.5. As is evident from the figure, the more immunosuppressed the host organism, the less the inflammatory cellular infiltration of lesions. This is also true for the early phase of GvHD. Skin rash, macroscopically visible at this time, may primarily result from a vascular reaction induced by cytokines. Thereafter, in a second phase, a sparse infiltration of lesions by T-lymphocytes, NK cells and monocytes/macrophages can be observed [120]. If scattered individual apoptotic keratinocytes additionally appear, the histomorphological picture is diagnostic of GvHD.

The inflammatory infiltrates present in GvHD lesions are very unusual insofar as they consist of a mixture of cells derived from two different individuals, donor and recipient. This cellular medley underlines impressively that the histomorphological manifestations of acute GvHD represent the result of a complex set of interacting variables [66].

3.6 Comparison of GvHR and HvGR

The striking difference between inflammation under the conditions of immunocompetence and immunodeficiency can also be demonstrated by a comparison of graft-versus-host reaction (GvHR) with host-versus-graft reaction (HvGR). First of all, one should remember that HvGR (allograft rejection), GvHR and inflammation are primarily mechanisms of defense. The purpose of these defense mechanisms is to distinguish between self and not-self [45] and to eliminate foreign cells or microbial pathogens [1]. However, like other physiological mechanisms, they may induce pathological reactions and tissue damage under certain conditions. This is likewise the case with HvGR and GvHR.

Allograft rejection and GvHD are "mirror images" [117]. This is true in several respects:

1. The likelihood of the manifestation in both correlates with the degree of genetic disparity between donor and recipient [117, 188].
2. Both allograft rejection and GvHD, in the HLA-identical setting, are mediated by alloreactive T-lymphocytes [117, 303].
3. Both can occur in acute and in chronic form [188].
4. The histomorphology of the two lesions shows a close similarity [76, 188, 202, 249].

However, there also are distinct differences: while the allogeneic T-lymphocytes in GvHD stem from the donor, in allograft rejection they are derived from the recipient. Whereas acute GvHD, e.g., of the liver, shows a purely lymphocytic infiltration, acute hepatic allograft rejection discloses a mixed infiltrate composed of lymphocytes, neutrophils, and eosinophils [76, 249]. This difference in histomorphology is not accidental but corresponds to profound differences in the immune state of the two types of patients. While patients developing acute GvHD are in most instances severely myelo- and immunosuppressed, patients experiencing acute allograft rejection are usually immunocompetent. Thus, in spite of many similarities there are distinct differences between allograft rejection and GvHD that have important implications for our understanding of the histomorphology of acute GvHD.

3.7 Pathogenesis of Chronic GvHD

The pathogenesis of chronic GvHD is still largely unknown [149, 332]. Risk factors for the development of chronic GvHD are prior acute GvHD, pre-transplant conditioning, and the age of patients [184]. Thus, adults have a higher incidence and severity of chronic GvHD than children [159]. Infants with SCID, who receive no conditioning prior to HLA-identical HSCT, develop no or only transient acute GvHD and no chronic GvHD [105, 215]. Occasionally, viral infections of the skin may trigger chronic cutaneous GvHD [25]. Still, the most important risk factor for chronic GvHD is preceding acute GvHD [19, 27, 176, 184].

Most authors assume that chronic GvHD, like acute GvHD, is primarily induced by alloreactive donor T-lymphocytes [176, 304] and that it may be due largely to a covert or subclinical continuation of the acute disease [277]. Host-specific cytotoxic lymphocytes as well as IL-2-secreting T-helper cells are indeed present in the blood of patients with chronic GvHD [43, 171]. This is compatible with the observation that chronic GvHD lesions contain CD8$^+$ as well as CD4$^+$ T-lymphocytes [15]. If these T-cells are removed from allogeneic bone marrow transplants by monoclonal antibodies, the incidence of chronic GvHD is strongly reduced [68, 129, 130]. This indicates that alloreactive donor T-lymphocytes in fact do play a significant role in the pathogenesis of chronic GvHD. There is evidence that cytokines are involved also [255].

Chronic GvHD resembles autoimmune connective tissue disease in several respects [174, 285]. The pathogenetic sequence may start with damage to the thymus by pretransplant conditioning, by posttransplant GvHD prophylaxis with CSA, or by acute GvHD [219, 283]. This thymic damage might lead to disturbances of immunoregulation, humoral as well as cellular immuno-deficiency, and autoimmune tissue damage [19, 255]. It is not surprising that the serum of patients with chronic GvHD often contains a variety of autoantibodies [253, 255], and yet there is no direct correlation between the presence or level of these autoantibodies and the development of chronic GvHD [70, 71]. Consequently, such autoantibodies possess neither pathogenetic nor diagnostic significance [176]. In contrast, autoreactive T-cells do play an important role in the collagen deposition that is characteristic of chronic GvHD [242]. Altogether, chronic GvHD represents a multiorgan syndrome with alloimmune and autoimmune features [64, 283].

4 Clinical Manifestations of GvHD

GvHD, as outlined before, can occur in a number of different clinical situations and under different pathogenetic conditions. However, GvHD most frequently is observed in the setting of allogeneic HSCT. These patients, almost without exception, receive some kind of immunosuppressive GvHD prophylaxis (Table 3.1) after transplantation [75, 200, 245, 306, 350]. Therefore, today, the clinical features of GvHD often are modified by pretransplant conditioning and posttransplant prophylaxis [75, 200].

As far as HLA-identical sibling HSCT is concerned, the incidence of GvHD has decreased, the onset is postponed and the clinical manifestations are mitigated. Nowadays, atypical forms of GvHD occur more frequently. The diagnosis of GvHD, clinically as well as histologically, has not been made easier by this change, on the contrary it has been rendered more difficult. Nevertheless, patients showing signs of GvHD without pretransplant conditioning and posttransplant GvHD prophylaxis still occur. This holds true for TA-GvHD [10, 124], for GvHD after allogeneic HSCT for SCID [103, 104, 105, 113], and for patients receiving allogeneic DLI [182]. In addition, the increased use of alternative donors has led to a situation in which cases of severe GvHD can still be observed [52].

4.1 Clinical Features of Acute GvHD

Acute GvHD develops in about 30%–60% of recipients of histocompatible sibling HSCT [16]. From the foregoing discussion it is evident that the conditions for the manifestation of GvHD today are much more variable than they were 10 or 20 years ago. Acute GvHD occurs today not only immediately after allogeneic HSCT but also at any later time when posttransplant immunosuppression is discontinued, e. g., after withdrawal of CSA for leukemia relapse [90].

After allogeneic HSCT, acute GvHD usually develops within 2–6 weeks [70], the median onset being about 3 weeks [255]. If no immunosuppression is given or if HLA-nonidentical bone marrow is used [255], hyperacute GvHD can manifest within about 8 days [305, 307]. The hyperacute syndrome is characterized by fever, fluid retention, severe skin disease, and a variable involvement of liver and gut [70]. An accelerated onset may also be observed in TA-GvHD [10, 301] or after second HSCT subsequent to allograft rejection [315]. Primary targets of acute GvHD are skin, liver, and GIT. In addition, the lymphatic organs (immune system), bone marrow, mucous membranes, and mucosa of the respiratory tract may be affected.

4.1.1 Acute GvHD of the Skin

The skin is the organ most frequently (>90%) affected by acute GvHD. A maculopapular rash, often involving the face, palms, and soles, is commonly the first manifestation (Fig. 4.1). This distribution is characteristic and of diagnostic significance [70, 120]. Subsequently the rash can spread over the chest, shoulders, abdomen, and finally involve the entire body (Fig. 4.2). In most cases the rash is diffuse, but occasionally it has a punctate appearance indicating a predominant involvement of the hair follicles [120].

The clinical symptoms of acute GvHD of the skin vary considerably. Frequently, patients complain of pruritus and burning palms or soles. If there is a localized rash only, it may cause few symptoms and disappear without treatment. In moderately acute GvHD up to half of the body surface is involved, in severe GvHD the entire body. While clinical symptoms in the former case are mostly mild, they are marked if erythroderma is generalized, with bulla formation, epidermal necrosis, exfoliation, or denudation of the skin as seen after severe burns (Fig. 4.3).

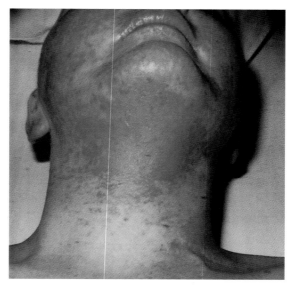

Fig. 4.1. Acute GvHD of skin. Confluent maculopapular rash of face and neck. 36-year-old female patient with MDS 42 days after HLA-identical allogeneic BMT

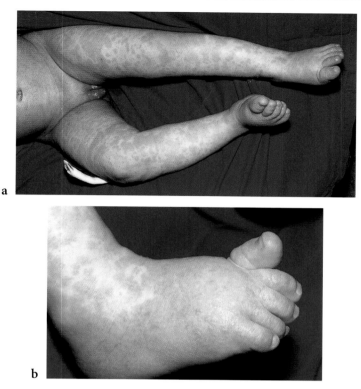

Fig. 4.2 a, b. Acute GvHD of skin. Maculopapular rash involving the entire body surface. **a** Overview. **b** Close view. $1^3/_4$-year-old female infant with MHC class II-deficiency 35 days after HLA-nonidentical allogeneic BMT

Acute GvHD of skin usually is a clinical diagnosis [255], but sometimes the distinction from conditioning-induced skin damage is clinically difficult. In this situation a skin biopsy can be helpful [19, 70, 255]. In contrast, the determination of serum levels of cytokines or of other humoral parameters, does not at present reliably distinguish acute GvHD from toxic skin damage [108, 125, 139, 179]. This may change in the future.

4.1.2 Acute GvHD of the Liver

In approximately 40%–60% of patients with acute GvHD the liver is involved. Hepatic lesions usually manifest somewhat later than the skin disease, within 3–6 weeks after allogeneic HSCT [255]. Isolated acute GvHD of liver without involvement of the skin is rare. Clinical manifestation of hepatic GvHD prior to skin GvHD is also uncommon [123, 321].

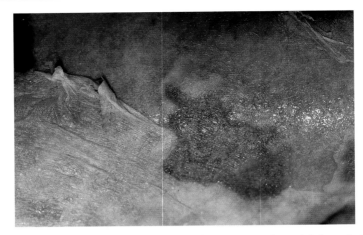

Fig. 4.3. Acute GvHD of skin with epidermal necrosis and partial denudation. Post mortem finding in a 43-year-old female patient with CML 29 days after HLA-identical unrelated allogeneic BMT. Acute GvHD of liver present simultaneously

The clinical symptoms of acute hepatic GvHD are quite unspecific [63]. Patients may complain of abdominal pain and show jaundice, liver enlargement, and ascites [255]. Usually the liver damage becomes evident by rising serum levels of bilirubin, alkaline phosphatase, and aspartate aminotransferase [70]. Sometimes γ-glutamyltranspeptidase titers are also elevated.

There are a number of other causes of hepatic dysfunction after allogeneic HSCT, such as conditioning-induced toxicity, venoocclusive disease (VOD) and viral hepatitis, which all can be difficult to distinguish from GvHD [63, 87]. Since neither the clinical picture nor the biochemical profile in the posttransplant phase is specific, a liver biopsy may be helpful. In most instances, a distinction between GvHD and other HSCT-associated liver complications will be possible histologically [286]. However, if hepatic dysfunction develops in a patient with unequivocal skin and/or gastrointestinal GvHD a liver biopsy is not needed.

4.1.3 Acute GvHD of the Gastrointestinal Tract

Acute gastrointestinal GvHD develops in about 30%–50% of allogeneic BMT recipients [56]. Involvement of the GIT is of utmost prognostic significance [86, 146] since the mortality of severe forms of gastrointestinal GvHD may reach 30%–60% [56]. Clinically, it manifests itself at the same time as or shortly after the onset of cutaneous GvHD [216]. Isolated GvHD of the GIT is rare. Gut manifestation before skin disease also is uncommon

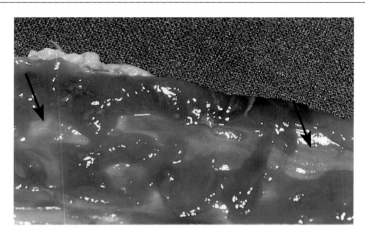

Fig. 4.4. Acute GvHD of gut with extensive ulcerations of the colonic mucosa (*arrow*). Post mortem finding in a 10-month-old male infant with SCID 14 days after transfusion of non-irradiated blood. Severe acute GvHD of skin present simultaneously

[123, 321]. Basically, all parts of the GIT can be affected [216], although lesions appear to be more frequent and aggressive in the distal ileum and proximal colon than in the upper GIT [112]. This may reflect the distribution of bacterial flora [216]. Endoscopically, manifestations of acute GvHD vary from subtle mucosal erythema and edema to enterocolitis with frank ulceration and denudation (Fig. 4.4).

Clinical symptoms of patients with acute GvHD of the GIT are anorexia, nausea, vomiting, abdominal pain, and diarrhea which may become bloody if the disease progresses [255, 293]. In severe cases a paralytic ileus, recognizable by X-ray, may develop [273]. All clinical symptoms are nonspecific and of limited diagnostic value [261, 298]. Within the first 20–25 days after allogeneic HSCT the differential diagnosis of acute GvHD includes chemoradiation toxicity and opportunistic infections of the intestine. Patients with upper gastrointestinal GvHD frequently also have extensive skin GvHD [261]. When the symptoms point to the lower GIT (e. g., diarrhea) endoscopy with colorectal biopsy is indicated. In general, biopsies taken more than 20–25 days after transplantation permit histological recognition of acute GvHD [298, 348].

4.1.4 Acute GvHD of Other Organs

Under certain conditions there are a number of other GvHD target organs that may acquire considerable clinical and prognostic significance. The bone marrow, for instance, can be damaged severely by TA-GvHD [10]. While in patients with allogeneic BMT the bone marrow is not normally a target for GvHD, since both the hematopoietic cells and the T-cells are of donor origin, in patients with TA-GvHD the T-lymphocytes are of donor and the hematopoietic cells of host origin [41, 133], and therefore alloreactive donor T-cells can attack and destroy the bone marrow of the recipient. Consequently, bone marrow failure, pancytopenia, and a rapidly fatal course are characteristic of TA-GvHD [10].

Another important target of acute GvHD is the immune system, in particular the thymus [219]. GvHD-induced lesions in the thymus may cause long-lasting immunodeficiency, a major factor in morbidity and mortality after allogeneic HSCT.

Whether acute GvHD can damage the lungs has been a subject of debate from the very beginning. In the early years various pulmonary alterations, such as restrictive or obstructive ventilatory changes, were interpreted clinically as manifestations of acute GvHD of the lung. However, histomorphologically no lesions characteristic of acute GvHD could be identified [292, 300]. More recently evidence has been advanced that the lung in fact can be involved by GvHD [351], and that the mucosal epithelium of bronchi and bronchioli might be a target for the alloimmune attack [277]. On the other hand, most of the pulmonary diseases that occur in some 40%–60% of patients after allogeneic HSCT, and which contribute significantly to the morbidity and mortality of such patients, are obviously caused by other pathogenetic factors such as viral infections or chemoradiation toxicity [22].

Finally, a large number of organ and tissue changes have been interpreted clinically as manifestations of acute GvHD. To the present there is no direct proof for such assumptions.

4.1.5 Clinical Grading of Acute GvHD

To determine the clinical severity of acute GvHD and to predict the posttransplant outcome of patients, Glucksberg et al. [123] designed a grading system, revised by Thomas et al. [321]. This Glucksberg-Thomas or Glucksberg-Seattle scoring is based on the separate assessment of the clinical severity of pathological changes in the three major GvHD target organs skin, liver, and intestine (Table 4.1). The changes observed are then used for clinical grading of acute GvHD (Table 4.2). This grading system has been successfully used over many years all over the world [70].

Within the past 10 years Glucksberg-Thomas scoring, possibly due to changes in donor selection, transplantation modalities, and/or GvHD prophylaxis, has proved to be no longer completely satisfactory [255]. Attempts have consequently been made to improve the clinical grading of acute GvHD [73, 251]. In addition, the International Bone Marrow Transplantation Registry (IBMTR) proposed a new GvHD severity index not requiring sub-

Table 4.1. Clinical severity of organ involvement by acute GvHD (modified from Glucksberg et al. [123], Thomas et al. [321], Rowlings et al. [260])

Stage	Skin	Liver	Gastrointestinal tract
1	Maculopapular rash <25% of body surface	Bilirubin 34–50 μmol/l	Diarrhea 500–1000 ml/day
2	Maculopapular rash <25% of body surface	Bilirubin 51–102 μmol/l	Diarrhea 1000–1500 ml/day
3	Generalized erythroderma	Bilirubin 103–225 μmol/l	Diarrhea >1500 ml/day
4	Generalized erythroderma with bullous formation and desquamation	Bilirubin >225 μmol/l	Severe abdominal pain, with or without ileus

Table 4.2. Clinical grading of acute GvHD (modified from Glucksberg et al. [123], Thomas et al. [321], Rowlings et al. [260])

Grade	Skin	Liver	Gastrointestinal tract	Clinical performance
I	1–2 [a]	0	0	No decrease
II	1–3	1	1	Mild decrease
III	2–3	2–3	2–3	Marked decrease
IV	2–4	2–4	2–4	Extreme decrease

[a] Stage of individual organ involvement, see Table 4.1.

jective clinical assessment [260]. When the IBMTR severity index was tested, some investigators found the index more predictive than the Glucksberg-Thomas criteria [207], whereas others found it had no advantage[205, 206]. It appears that any method used for grading of acute GvHD has advantages and disadvantages and none is perfect.

There are several points that still need to be made:

1. Lack of satisfaction with the different clinical scoring systems has led to a proposal for retrospective grading of acute GvHD whereby the response to therapy and the outcome determine the final grade [70].
2. The obvious insufficiency of clinical criteria to predict the posttransplant outcome suggests that it might be worthwhile to test the prognostic potential of histological criteria.

3. Up to the present there is no indication that a blood test or some other clinical measure can take over the diagnostic function of a biopsy.
4. The importance of grading acute GvHD is evident if one notes that survival directly correlates with GvHD severity grade: > 90 % in grade I, about 60 % in grade II-III, almost 0 % in grade IV [334].

4.2 Clinical Features of Chronic GvHD

Chronic GvHD is a pleiotropic syndrome resembling autoimmune connective tissue disorders. It possesses considerable variability in mode of onset, organs involved, and rate of progression [285]. Chronic GvHD occurs in 30 % – 50 % of recipients of HLA-identical sibling BMT [19, 63, 73, 159, 255].

The most important risk factor for chronic GvHD is prior acute GvHD [19, 27]. Its incidence after HLA-identical sibling transplantation is age-dependent: 13 % in children < 10 years, 28 % in adolescents 10 – 19 years, and 42 % – 46 % in adults > 20 years [174]. Chronic GvHD may occur more often after PBSCT than after BMT [61, 282, 304]. The prophylactic use of CSA, MTX, and other immunosuppressants has reduced the incidence and severity of acute GvHD but has not diminished problems caused by chronic GvHD [16, 75, 334].

The outcome of chronic GvHD depends on patient age, type of onset, severity, and course of the disease. Chronic GvHD in adults usually is more severe and prognosis is worse than in children [159]. The overall mortality is high [128, 296]. Most deaths do not result from direct failure of the GvHD target organs but from infections promoted by GvHD-associated immunodeficiency [64, 332].

The onset of chronic GvHD varies considerably [15, 71, 176, 285]:

1. It may develop as a continuation of acute GvHD, so-called progressive type (ca. 32 % of cases).
2. It may follow acute GvHD after a variable symptom free period, so-called quiescent type (ca. 36 % of cases).
3. It may occur without evidence of prior acute GvHD, so-called de novo type (ca. 30 % of cases).

The prognosis of patients with chronic GvHD of the progressive type is worst, of the quiescent type is intermediate, and of the de novo type is best [176, 305].

The spectrum of target organs of chronic GvHD is much larger and more variable than that of acute GvHD [176, 255, 277, 305, 306]. The three classical target organs skin, liver, and GIT again play a major role in chronic GvHD.

4.2.1 Chronic GvHD of the Skin

The skin is the organ most frequently involved. It is affected in 80% – 90% of patients with chronic GvHD [15, 77, 176, 253, 334]. Chronic cutaneous GvHD may develop slowly after allogeneic HSCT, or may develop rapidly, e.g., if immunosuppression is discontinued [255]. The skin manifestations are either localized (20% of patients) or generalized (80% of patients [176, 219, 277, 284]). Clinically as well as histologically two different types of lesions can be distinguished: lichenoid lesions, starting early, that is, about 3 months after transplantation; and sclerodermatous lesions, occurring at a later time, that is, 6 – 12 months posttransplantation [19, 176].

Lichenoid Type

The lichenoid variant (Fig. 4.5) is characterized by violaceous papules showing a lichen planus-like appearance, and frequently starting at the distal parts of the extremities [176]. Clinical symptoms are itching and dryness of skin as a consequence of reduced sweat production [176]. In addition to the lichenoid papules there are areas of erythema and/or dyspigmentation [255]. Occasionally, local hyper- or hypopigmentation can be the sole clinical manifestation of chronic GvHD [255].

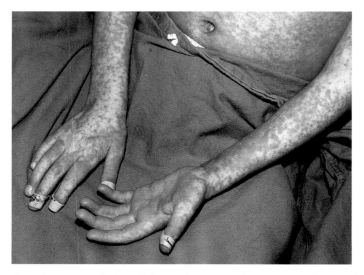

Fig. 4.5. Chronic GvHD of skin, lichenoid type. Violaceous papules involving the entire body surface. A 15-year-old male patient with AML 12 months after HLA-non-identical allogeneic BMT. Chronic GvHD of GIT present simultaneously

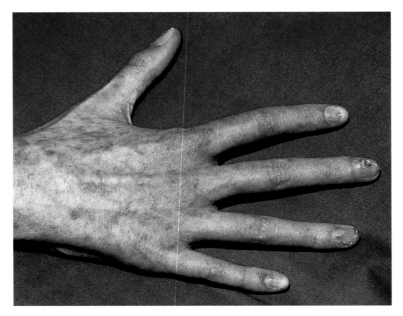

Fig. 4.6. Chronic GvHD of skin with nail dystrophy. Same patient as in Fig. 4.5

Sclerodermatous Type

The sclerodermatous variant is characterized by a sclerotic dermis, atrophic epidermis, and dyspigmentation [176, 277]. Clinically, the generalized form closely resembles scleroderma, the localized form morphea [277]. Severe chronic GvHD of skin may be associated with nail dystrophy (Fig. 4.6), alopecia, and formation of bullae and ulcers [19, 176].

4.2.2 Chronic GvHD of the Liver

The liver is affected in approximately 30% of patients with chronic GvHD [253]. Almost all of these patients also have chronic GvHD of skin. The hepatic lesions can be either part of an extensive chronic GvHD involving many organs or it may be part of a more limited disease involving the skin and liver only [176]. Isolated hepatic GvHD without involvement of any other organ is extremely rare.

Clinically, patients frequently show obstructive jaundice caused by damage to the small intrahepatic bile ducts [255]. It is noteworthy that chronic GvHD of the liver and primary biliary cirrhosis (PBC) have many clinical and laboratory features in common [253, 287]. This holds true, for example, for the autoantibodies occurring in serum of both groups of patients. Also, as a consequence of the GvHD-induced damage to the biliary system, patients may show a marked increase in serum alkaline phosphatase levels, a finding by no means pathognomonic for hepatic GvHD. A liver biopsy can be useful in settling the differential diagnosis.

4.2.3 Chronic GvHD of the Gastrointestinal Tract

Chronic gastrointestinal GvHD occurs much less frequently than acute GvHD of the GIT [293]. About 30% of patients with chronic GvHD show some kind of gastrointestinal involvement [253]. The mean posttransplant

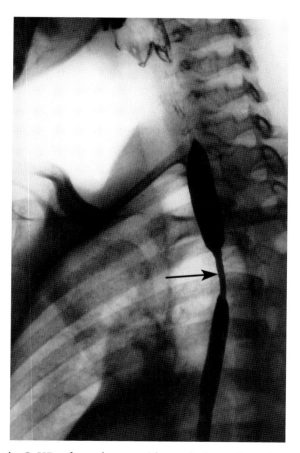

Fig. 4.7. Chronic GvHD of esophagus with marked esophageal stenosis (*arrow*). A 14-year-old female patient with FA 18 months after HLA-identical allogeneic BMT. Chronic GvHD of skin and liver present simultaneously

time for observation of lesions is 5.8 months with a range of 3–16 months [17]. In most patients the skin is also affected. An isolated involvement of the stomach or the intestines by chronic GvHD is rare.

The clinical symptoms of patients with chronic GvHD of the GIT such as diarrhea, malabsorption, or weight loss are nonspecific [176]. Patients occasionally complain of abdominal pain, anorexia, and nausea and vomiting [255]. Whereas chronic GvHD of the esophagus in earlier years developed frequently [211], with modern immunosuppressive treatment this manifestation has become rare [255]. Altogether chronic GvHD of the GIT in contrast to acute gastrointestinal GvHD plays only a minor clinical role.

4.2.4 Chronic GvHD of Other Organs

The spectrum of target organs of chronic GvHD is much larger than that of acute GvHD. Many other organs in addition to skin, liver, and GIT may be involved. To be noted is the sicca syndrome, which affects 80% of patients with chronic GvHD [277]. In this syndrome the mouth is involved in more than 70% of cases (Fig. 4.8), the eyes in up to 80% and the nose and/or the airways in a variable percentage [70, 176]. Also frequently affected by chronic GvHD are the immune and hematopoietic systems [133, 255] and the lungs [84, 240].

The consequences of damage to the lymphatic organs by chronic GvHD may be severe immunodeficiency, predisposing to recurrent potentially

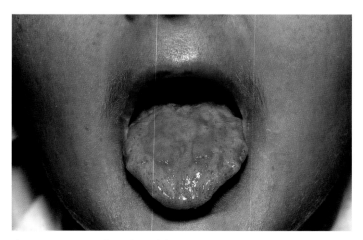

Fig. 4.8. Chronic GvHD of oral and lingual mucosa with epithelial hyperplasia. Icterus of skin due to hepatic involvement by chronic GvHD. Same patient as in Fig. 4.7

lethal infections [19, 255], or to autoimmune diseases such as polymyositis, myasthenia gravis, and many others [16, 277]. Hence, autoantibodies to smooth muscle, mitochondria, and other cellular components are frequently found in the serum of patients with chronic GvHD [176, 253, 255].

A long list of other pathological changes have been ascribed to chronic GvHD. However, often it is difficult or impossible to decide whether the respective tissue changes in fact are caused by chronic GvHD or by one of the numerous other pathogenetic mechanisms also active in patients after allogeneic HSCT [74].

4.2.5 Clinical Classification of Chronic GvHD

For the clinical grading of chronic GvHD different parameters are used. Basically, the disease may be subclinical (up to 30% of cases) or clinically overt (ca. 70% of cases), localized (ca. 20% of cases) or generalized (ca. 80% of cases), limited or extensive [277]. By these criteria a classification of chronic GvHD is possible (Table 4.3). As is evident from the table, the clinical evaluation alone is insufficient for the assessment of organs such as the liver or the salivary glands. Grading of the severity of chronic GvHD in these

Table 4.3. Clinicopathological classification of chronic GvHD (modified from Sullivan [305, 306], Klingemann [176])

Classification	Grade	Clinical or histological criteria
Subclinical	I	Clinically no GvHD evident, but histologically positive
Limited	II	Either or both: Localized skin involvement Hepatic dysfunction due to GvHD
Extensive	III	Either: Generalized skin involvement Or: Localized skin involvement and/or hepatic dysfunction due to GvHD plus: Liver histology showing chronic aggressive hepatitis, bridging necrosis, or cirrhosis; or Involvement of eye (Schirmer's test with <5 mm wetting); or Involvement of minor salivary glands or oral mucosa demonstrated on labial biopsy; or Involvement of any other target organ, e.g., lung

organs additionally requires a histomorphological investigation. Subclinical chronic GvHD also can only be assessed by skin or oral biopsy. Consequently, the clinical grading of chronic GvHD is a combined clinicopathological classification (Table 4.3) which has been found to be reproducible and to possess a considerable prognostic potential [176].

5 Histopathological Manifestations of Acute GvHD

A presentation of the histopathology of acute GvHD comprises three aspects:

1. A description of the morphological correlates of clinically manifest GvHD (clinical pathology)
2. A discussion of the diagnostic potential of biopsies for recognition of acute GvHD (diagnostic pathology)
3. A presentation of the histological critera for grading the severity of acute GvHD

As outlined before, GvHD lesions represent the end result of a highly complex interaction of multiple pathogenetic factors. Due to the dynamic nature of this process, the histological picture of GvHD lesions is not constant and stereotyped but changes with time and environmental conditions. Pretransplant preparation and posttransplant GvHD prophylaxis can modify the immune response and the inflammatory reaction, and, thus, the histological picture considerably. It is not an exaggeration to say that under today's conditions the pathologist gets to see only that part of GvHD not suppressed by GvHD prophylaxis. This is illustrated schematically in Fig. 5.1. Without

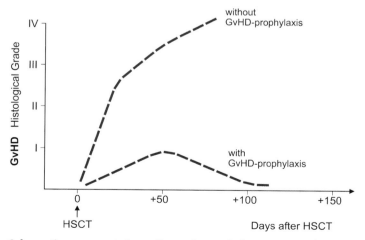

Fig. 5.1. Schematic representation of severity and time course of acute GvHD in patients with or without immunosuppressive GvHD prophylaxis

immunosuppressive GvHD prophylaxis, many patients develop severe acute GvHD after allogeneic HSCT (Fig. 5.1, *upper curve*) and may die. In contrast, if GvHD prophylaxis is provided most patients suffer only mild acute GvHD (Fig. 5.1, *lower curve*) and survive. Today the latter course is seen much more frequently. Nowadays, the histopathology of GvHD, with a few exceptions, is a histomorphology under the influence of immunosuppressive GvHD prophylaxis.

The situation is paradoxical, however. GvHD prophylaxis not only reduces the incidence and severity of GvHD but may itself cause lesions that in fact resemble GvHD.

If these considerations are taken into account, it is not surprising that opinions concerning the value of biopsy in the diagnosis of GvHD range from important and reliable [19, 205, 206, 208, 277] to useless and unreliable [24, 227, 294, 352]. While authors espousing the latter opinion claim that the histomorphology of GvHD cannot be distinguished from other lesions, those in the former camp regard GvHD histopathology as valid, in fact a conditio sine qua non for the diagnosis of GvHD. So what is the truth? The following presentation should give an answer to this question.

Since acute GvHD after allogeneic HSCT, as compared to GvHD following blood transfusion, materno-fetal transfusion, or solid organ transplantation, plays by far the most important role, we will concentrate primarily but not exclusively on post-HSCT GvHD. This focus of attention is justified by the fact that the histomorphological picture of acute GvHD occurring in different clinical situations is basically comparable. Any exceptions to this rule will be pointed out.

As discussed previously, the major targets of acute GvHD are skin, liver, and GIT. Sometimes, too, lymphatic organs, bone marrow, mucous membranes, and airways are affected. Since acute GvHD most often starts in the skin, since the skin is more frequently involved than any other organ, since skin biopsies are less likely to result in clinical complications than biopsies from liver or GIT, and since they can be initially taken and repeated without difficulty, skin biopsies possess by far the greatest significance in the histomorphological assessment of acute GvHD [120, 272, 277, 288, 289].

5.1 Histological Features of Acute GvHD of the Skin

The onset of acute GvHD after allogeneic HSCT depends on a number of factors. In general, the greater the antigenic disparity between donor and host, the sooner the onset of acute GvHD [288]. Also, the more severe the acute GvHD, the earlier the appearance of cutaneous lesions [162].

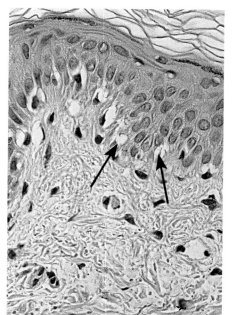 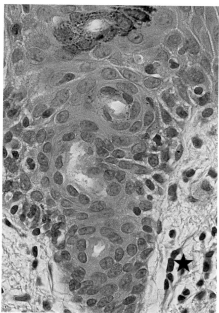

a   b

Fig. 5.2a, b. Early low-grade histological changes in acute GvHD of the skin. Focal vacuolization of basal cells (*arrows*). Scanty lymphocytic infiltration of the papillary dermis (*asterisk*). **a** Biopsy of an 8-year-old male patient with AML obtained 9 days after HLA-identical allogeneic BMT. The child 10 days later displayed overt acute GvHD of the skin, liver, and GIT. **b** Biopsy of a 14-year-old male patient with AA taken 10 days after HLA-identical related allogeneic BMT. Lateron the patient developed chronic cutaneous and hepatic GvHD. H&E, ×420

5.1.1 Early Acute GvHD of the Skin

Early acute GvHD of the skin, macroscopically evident by a rash 2–3 weeks after allogeneic HSCT, histologically shows focal basal cell vacuolization of the epidermis and, sometimes, a slight perivascular lymphocytic infiltration of the upper dermis (Fig. 5.2; [120, 208, 277]). These trifling early changes are histologically nonspecific and cannot be safely distinguished from cutaneous damage induced by pretransplant chemoradiation conditioning [272, 311]. Histomorphologically they correspond to the initial "endothelial phase" of cutaneous delayed-type hypersensitivity reactions in which there is endothelial activation with consecutive early T-cell influx into the papillary dermis, not the epidermis [120]. Such lesions cannot be relied on for a sound histological diagnosis.

In addition, the early lesions of acute GvHD are often only focal and discrete. Biopsies taken immediately after onset of the rash are frequently

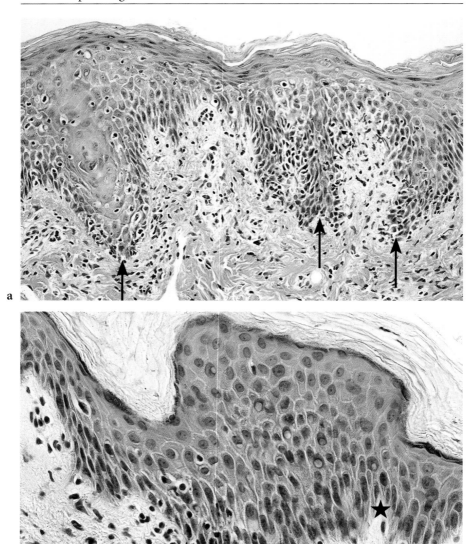

Fig. 5.3 a, b. Incipient acute GvHD of the skin. Sparse lymphocytic infiltration of the upper dermis with exocytosis of lymphocytes into the rete ridges of the tangentially cut epidermis (*arrows*). Melanin is still present in the basal layer (*asterisk*). **a** Biopsy of a 16-year-old male patient with AML obtained 11 weeks after HLA-identical unrelated allogeneic BMT. The patient subsequently developed overt acute GvHD of the skin and oral mucosa. **b** Biopsy of a 7-year-old female patient with FA obtained 10 days after HLA-identical unrelated allogeneic BMT. Shortly thereafter the child manifested acute GvHD of the skin and GIT. H & E, **a** ×210, **b** ×328

falsely negative [144]. In contrast, biopsies obtained 24–48 h later are more likely to show tissue changes histologically compatible with acute GvHD [88]. This, for instance, can be a lymphocytic infiltration of the rete ridges in lesional skin (Fig. 5.3). Such lymphocytic infiltrates at the dermo-epidermal junction are diagnostically important because they are the harbinger of target-cell injury, that is, individual keratinocyte apoptosis.

GvHD is treated most effectively when detected early [168]. In the early phase, therapeutic intervention can prevent progression to higher-grade disease and thus improve the outcome [180, 291]. Unfortunately, as stated previously, there is a time lag between the clinical onset of the skin rash and the histological appearance of lymphocytic infiltrates in lesional skin [325]. Most authors agree that a reliable histological diagnosis of acute GvHD cannot be made in the absence of an epidermal lymphocytic infiltration [88, 154, 208, 234, 288].

5.1.2 Established Acute GvHD of the Skin

About 3–6 weeks after transplantation GvHD skin lesions show a characteristic histomorphological picture. The epidermis is thinned and may focally exhibit spongiosis. There is a sprinkling of lymphocytes along the dermo-epidermal junction and scattered damaged ("dyskeratotic") keratinocytes in the basal or suprabasal layers of the epidermis [168]. Some of these damaged keratinocytes appear as pale round coreless discs, others as eosinophilic bodies (Fig. 5.4).

Occasionally, lymphocytes surround an individual damaged keratinocyte, a phenomenon called "satellitosis" (Fig. 5.5). Satellitosis is very characteristic of acute GvHD but is detectable in only about 24% of cases [208]. Therefore, it is by no means an absolute requirement for the histological diagnosis of GvHD. The upper dermis of lesions contains a perivascular or lichenoid lymphocytic infiltrate of variable density. Both the inflammatory infiltrate and the epidermal damage concentrate at the dermo-epidermal interface. From the point of view of the dermatopathologist, acute GvHD can hence be classified as interface dermatitis [3, 341]. In fact, the histomorphological substrate of established acute GvHD of the skin essentially is a lymphocytic interface dermatitis with individual damaged keratinocytes. The lesion corresponds to the "epidermotropic and target cell phase" of cutaneous GvHD as described by Gilliam and Murphy [120].

The inflammatory infiltrate in acute GvHD may include single eosinophils but usually no neutrophils. Macrophages, sometimes containing melanin, are also frequently present. Since the inflammatory infiltrate shows a predilection for the rete ridges of the epidermis and the parafollicular bulges of the hair follicles, some authors assume that the epithelial stem cells, located in these regions, are the primary target of acute GvHD [208, 269,

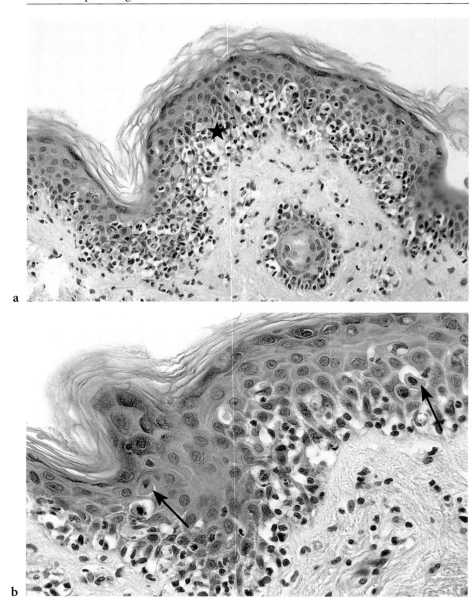

Fig. 5.4a, b. Established acute GvHD of the skin. Full blown lymphocytic interface dermatitis (*asterisk*). Multiple eosinophilic bodies (*arrows*). Biopsy of a 13-year-old male patient with ALL (acute lymphoblastic leukemia) obtained 31 days after HLA-identical allogeneic BMT. The patient also showed acute GvHD of the liver and GIT. H&E, **a** ×210, **b** ×328

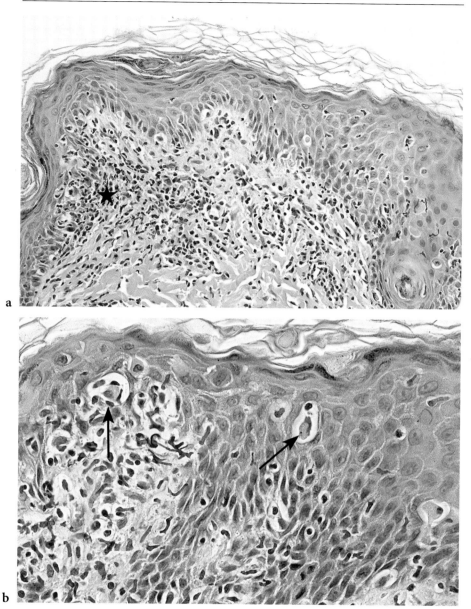

Fig. 5.5a, b. Established acute GvHD of the skin. Lymphocytic dermatitis focally obscuring the dermo-epidermal junction (*asterisk*). Multiple eosinophilic keratino-cytes with satellitosis (*arrows*). Biopsy of a 10-month-old infant with SCID obtained 9 weeks after HLA-identical related allogeneic BMT without pretransplant condition-ing. H & E, **a** × 210, **b** × 420

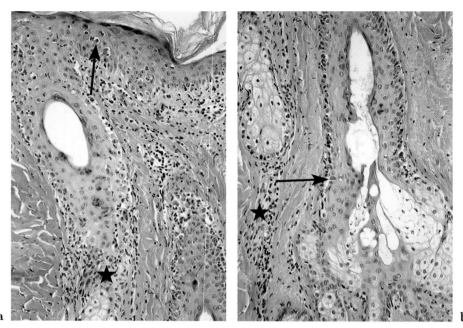

a   b

Fig. 5.6a, b. Acute GvHD of the skin with involvement of a pilosebaceous unit. Lymphocytic infiltration of epithelial structures (*asterisks*) and presence of multiple eosinophilic bodies (*arrows*). Biopsy of a 35-year-old female patient with AML obtained 24 days after HLA-identical allogeneic BMT. H & E, **a, b** × 120

275, 277]. This is in agreement with the observation that the hair follicles are affected in 57% – 100% of cases [55]. A typical pilosebaceous manifestation of acute GvHD is shown in Fig. 5.6.

Inflammatory Infiltrates in Acute GvHD

An important area of controversy in respect to the histomorphology of acute GvHD is the inflammatory infiltrate [311]. While some clinicians believe that acute GvHD may develop and can be diagnosed without an inflammatory infiltrate, most pathologists do not. In general pathologists are convinced that lymphocytes represent an integral component of GvHD lesions without which the histomorphological diagnosis cannot be made [154, 208, 234]. There are three obvious reasons for this controversy:

1. The amount of damage to the epidermis in acute GvHD is often out of proportion to the inflammatory infiltrate, which frequently is sparse [120, 197]. However, as previously discussed in detail, the almost universally

employed GvHD prophylaxis prevents the inflammatory infiltrate from being strong [277].

2. Skin biopsies in acute GvHD often are taken as early as possible, to wit, immediately after the onset of the skin rash.Quite obviously at this time a lymphocytic infiltration of skin, detectable by routine histology, is not yet present.

3. Although the requirement of alloreactive T-lymphocytes for the induction of acute GvHD is generally agreed, in recent years it has become increasingly clear that cytokines also are important effectors of acute GvHD. The erythema grossly visible at the onset of acute GvHD, at least in part, may be due to the action of cytokines. If this holds true, it appears logical that in the absence of epidermal lymphocytes one cannot histologically diagnose. But one also cannot histologically exclude early acute GvHD [311].

Overall, there is good evidence that the lymphocytic infiltrate, whether sparse or dense, in fact is an integral component of GvHD lesions. By in situ hybridization (ISH) of skin biopsies from patients after allogeneic sex-mismatched BMT or liver transplantation with Y-chromosome-specific probes, it has been shown that up to 90% of the lymphocytes present in lesions are of the donor genotype [20, 156]. This indicates that allogeneic lymphocytes of the donor are a major component of GvHD lesions.

These observations are substantiated by findings indicating that alloreactive donor T-lymphocytes in situ are required for the full development of GvHD lesions. This is evident from Y-chromosome-specific ISH showing that the number of donor lymphocytes in skin lesions correlates with the manifestation of GvHD: while early lesions contain only a few donor cells, in fully established GvHD the majority of lymphocytes are of the donor genotype [156]. Since other authors have shown that these in situ localized allogeneic donor T-lymphocytes possess host-specific cytotoxicity [118], there is little doubt that their presence in situ is needed for the full development of acute GvHD.

Cell Death in Acute GvHD

A second area of controversy in the histomorphology of acute GvHD is the nature and diagnostic significance of what pathologists formerly termed "dyskeratosis" [168]. Many other terms have been used for the cytopathic changes observed in acute GvHD, as seen in Table 5.1. The vast number of mostly descriptive and partially contradictory terms indicates the existing uncertainty. More recently it has become clear that true dyskeratosis, which in the strict sense means premature keratinization, is not increased in acute GvHD [3, 193]. In addition, it has been observed that most of the "dyskeratotic" keratinocytes in fact are dying or dead cells [168].

Table 5.1. Terms used in the literature to describe epithelial cell death in GvHD

"Dyskeratosis"	Eosinophilic body
"Dyskeratotic" keratinocyte	Acidophilic body
"Dyskeratotic" body	Colloid or hyalin body
Individual cell necrosis	Karyolytic body
Mummified cell	Apoptotic cell
Shrinkage necrosis	Apoptotic body
Granular necrosis	Apoptosis

Finally it has been shown that the mode of keratinocyte death in acute GvHD is apoptosis [193].

Apoptosis or programmed (active) cell death occurs in a wide variety of tissues, under physiological as well as pathological conditions [119]. It can be distinguished from nonprogrammed (passive, accidental) cell death as follows:

1. Apoptosis is characterized by shrinkage of the cell, condensation of nuclear chromatin, degradation of DNA, and fragmentation of nuclei, rapid phago-cytosis of apoptotic bodies, and lack of inflammatory reaction in tissue.
2. Nonprogrammed cell death or simple cell necrosis is characterized by swelling of the cell, release of lysosomal enzymes, nuclear digestion, and a distinct inflammatory reaction in tissue. By routine histology apoptosis and simple cell necrosis often are difficult to distinguish [168].

The occurrence of apoptotic keratinocytes in the presence of epidermotropic lymphocytic infiltrates is characteristic of acute GvHD of skin [168, 208]. Within these lesions the number of apoptotic keratinocytes correlates with the number of intraepidermal lymphocytes, in particular CD8+ T-cells [168, 173]. Whereas the scattered damaged keratinocytes are easily recognized in routine histology (Fig. 5.7a), specific identification of apoptosis is possible only by the TUNEL histochemical staining reaction (Fig. 5.7b [119]). As is evident from the figure, only part of the damaged keratinocytes exhibit a positive TUNEL staining. This might mean that not all of the respective keratinocytes show programmed cell death but rather simple cell necrosis or nonlethal damage. A reflection on the situation suggests that the additional occurrence of simple cell necrosis is a likely possibility, particularly in higher grade GvHD lesions.

Thus, the histomorphological hallmarks of acute cutaneous GvHD are single cell apoptosis of keratinocytes associated with intraepidermal lympho-cytic infiltrates. There may also be vacuolar degeneration of the basal layers of the epidermis, satellitosis, and a perivascular or lichenoid lymphocytic infil-tration of the upper dermis. All these pathological changes are focused on the

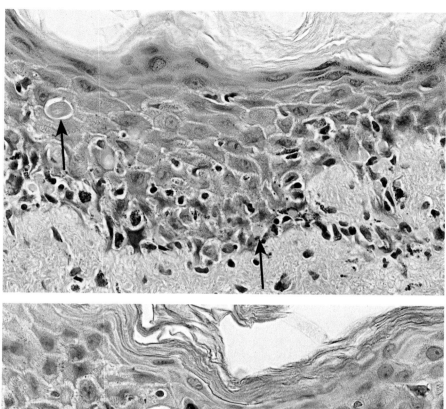

a

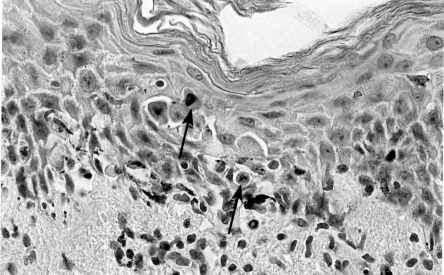

b

Fig. 5.7 a, b. Identification of apoptosis in acute cutaneous GvHD by TUNEL histo-chemical staining reaction. **a** In the H&E-staining several eosinophilic bodies are recognizable (*arrows*). **b** In the TUNEL staining a positive reaction of some of these eosinophilic (apoptotic) bodies is visible (*arrows*). **a, b** Biopsy of a 16-year-old male patient with CML and HLA-identical allogeneic BMT obtained 28 days after HLA-identical allogeneic DLI. **a** H&E, **b** TUNEL staining, kindly provided by Dr. J. Sträter, Ulm; **a, b** ×420

dermo-epidermal interface. The histomorphology of these lesions, at least qualitatively, does not depend on pretransplant conditioning since it is also present in TA-GvHD occurring in unconditioned patients [10, 124].

5.1.3 Severity of Acute GvHD of the Skin

The onset, severity, and course of acute GvHD in each individual patient is different, depending on factors such as clinical context of GvHD development, transplant modalities, and GvHD prophylaxis. Acute cutaneous GvHD may occur subclinically or may include only a transient, localized, spontaneously disappearing, mild skin rash. On the other hand it can manifest as a generalized rash persisting over long periods of time and histologically disclosing severe tissue changes.

To assess the severity of skin lesions a histological grading system was devised by Lerner et al. a long time ago [197]. This scoring system is exclusively based on the severity of damage to the epidermis:

Grade I: Mild changes, characterized by focal or diffuse vacuolar degeneration of epidermal basal cells and acanthocytes (Fig. 5.8a)

Grade II: Moderate changes, characterized by focal or diffuse spongiosis and eosinophilic degeneration (apoptosis) of scattered individual epidermal cells (Fig. 5.8b)

Grade III: Severe changes, characterized by separation of the dermo-epidermal junction and formation of clefts (Fig. 5.8c)

Grade IV: Maximal changes, characterized by extensive destruction and frank loss of epidermis (Fig. 5.8d)

Since the Lerner scoring system does not take into account the inflammatory infiltrate, which is an important diagnostic criterion, the histological parameters used for grading are not identical with those used for diagnosing acute GvHD. This issue has previously been discussed in detail. It is evident that neither very mild nor very severe lesions are diagnostic. Yet there is no doubt

Fig. 5.8a–d. Histological grading of acute GvHD of the skin. **a** Grade I = mild nonspecific changes of the epidermis. Single lymphocytes at the dermo-epidermal junction. **b** Grade II = moderate, histologically characteristic changes with lymphocytic infiltration of the epidermis and keratinocyte apoptosis. **c** Grade III = severe pathological changes with separation of the dermo-epidermal junction and cleft formation. **d** Grade IV = maximal changes with loss of epidermis and denudation. **a** Biopsy of the same patient as in Fig. 5.3b. **b** Biopsy of the same patient as in Fig. 5.6. **c** Biopsy of a 31-year-old female patient with AA obtained 31 days after allogeneic BMT. **d** Biopsy of a 4-week-old male infant with SCID, intrauterine MFT, and "exfoliative dermatitis" since birth. **a–d** H&E, **a–d** ×420

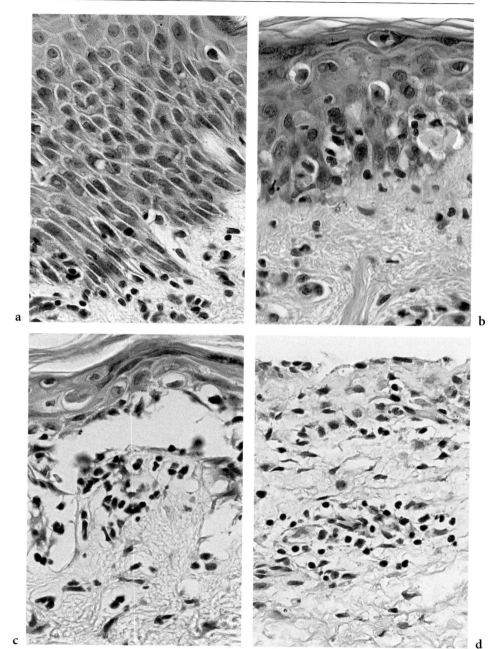

Fig. 5.8 a – d. Legend see p. 52

that the Lerner system, evaluating the severity of lesions in skin, liver, and gastrointestinal tract, possesses a significant prognostic potential [19].

5.1.4 Time Course of Acute GvHD of the Skin

The clinical course as well as the histomorphological picture of acute GvHD is profoundly influenced by GvHD prophylaxis and therapy (see Table 3.1 and Fig. 5.1 [70, 277, 302]). Withdrawal of CSA, MTX, or steroids from patients after allogeneic HSCT can result in late appearance or reappearance of florid GvHD lesions [327]. This indicates that GvHD may persist at a subclinical level after HSCT in patients receiving GvHD prophylaxis.

Overall, the influence of prophylactic and therapeutic measures on the course of acute GvHD is striking. Figure 5.9 illustrates a typical example as documented by follow-up biopsies, monitoring the response to therapy. As is evident from the figure, a prompt GvHD relapse occurs when prophylaxis with CSA/MTX is discontinued.

Depending on the severity of lesions and the efficacy of treatment, acute GvHD usually disappears within weeks or months. Frequently, the only residues histologically detectable are a slight atrophy of the epidermis, loss of

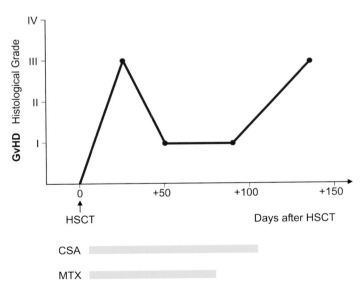

Fig. 5.9. Influence of GvHD prophylaxis on the course of acute GvHD of the skin as determined by follow-up biopsies (•) in a 28-year-old male patient with AML after HLA-identical unrelated allogeneic BMT. The first biopsy was taken 26 days after transplantation. Note prompt GvHD relapse after ending of GvHD prophylaxis. CSA, cyclosporine A; MTX, methotrexate

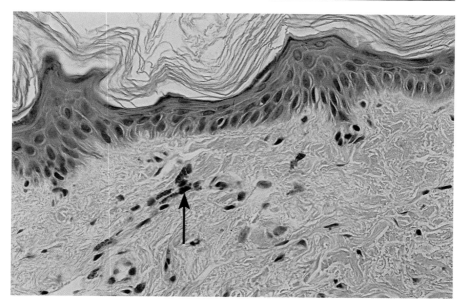

Fig. 5.10. Residual changes of the skin after healing of acute GvHD. There is slight atrophy of epidermis, hyperkeratosis, loss of pigment from the basal layer, and a focal accumulation of melanophages in the upper dermis (*arrow*). Biopsy of the same patient as in Fig. 5.3b, but taken 4 months after BMT. Condition of liver and GIT unremarkable. H & E, × 420

melanin from the stratum basale, and a focal accumulation of melanophages in the upper dermis (Fig. 5.10).

One other aspect needs to be mentioned: that is the poor correlation between the histomorphology of lesions and the clinical definition of acute or chronic GvHD. As a matter of fact, lesions showing the histological picture of acute GvHD have been observed in biopsies taken up to 481 days after allogeneic BMT [158, 327]. Therefore, the definition of acute and chronic GvHD by time range (acute GvHD = 0–100 days after BMT; chronic GvHD ≥ 100 days after BMT) does not correlate with the histopathological appearance of GvHD lesions. On the other hand, a purely histomorphological distinction of acute and chronic GvHD is feasible.

5.1.5 Histological Criteria of Acute GvHD of the Skin

Although specific pathognomonic criteria for the histological diagnosis of acute GvHD do not exist, and absolute certainty can never be achieved [94], there is a pattern of morphological phenomena consistent with the diagnosis of GvHD. As already delineated, the prime histological characteristics of acute GvHD of the skin are scattered individual apoptotic keratinocytes in conjunction with a variable, sometimes sparse lymphocytic infiltration at the dermo-epidermal interface and in the hair follicle epithelium [208]. The paucity of inflammatory infiltrates is due to the inability of most patients to recruit accessory cells into lesional skin in a normal fashion. This failure may be caused by a lack of such cells or a lack of cytokines to mobilize and direct them into the target area. Keratinocyte apoptosis with satellite lymphocytes (satellitosis) is present in a minor subgroup of lesions only [208]. As mentioned, satellitosis is a characteristic but not a consistent finding in acute GvHD.

Epidermal damage with single cell apoptosis suggestive of acute GvHD but lacking epidermotropic lymphocytic infiltration represents a possible diagnostic pitfall [136]. The histodiagnosis of acute GvHD is not feasible in the absence of an inflammatory infiltrate [88, 154, 208, 234]. Such a statement should be supplemented by adding that the infiltrate must be lymphocytic and must be localized intraepidermally. An exclusively dermal infiltration of lymphocytes has no discriminatory power at all [272].

Other histomorphological phenomena occuring in acute GvHD, such as vacuolization of basal cells, spongiosis, destruction of epidermis, or denudement, are not reliable histomorphological criteria for the diagnosis of acute GvHD. Nevertheless, they represent a safe basis for the widely used severity grading of GvHD [197, 272].

The clinical diagnosis of acute GvHD can be confirmed by histology if both epidermal damage and lymphocytic infiltration focused on the dermo-epidermal interface are present [288]. Lymphocytic infiltrates without epidermal damage or epidermal damage without inflammatory infiltration are insufficient criteria for the histological diagnosis of GvHD [158].

Advanced acute GvHD is easily recognized histologically. In contrast, early diagnosis of acute GvHD rarely is possible by routine histology. No single parameter such as keratinocyte apoptosis or satellitosis definitely proves the diagnosis of acute GvHD. Only the pattern of histomorphological phenomena described is characteristic of acute GvHD.

Similarly, single histomorphological criteria such as intraepithelial lymphocytes, apoptotic keratinocytes, pilosebaceous inflammation, follicular involvement, or dermal lymphocytic infiltration separately do not possess any prognostic significance [66]. In contrast, the combined parameters such as employed in the Lerner severity grading [197] have considerable prognostic potential [19].

5.1.6 Differential Diagnosis of Acute GvHD of the Skin

Unfortunately, the histomorphological features described are not unique to GvHD. There are a number of skin diseases that histologically resemble acute GvHD and therefore, theoretically, have to be considered in the differential diagnosis. This holds true for different types of interface dermatitis, contact dermatitis, erythema exsudativum multiforme, and discoid lupus erythematosus [3, 208, 277, 341]. Skin diseases such as lichen planus and psoriasis also show similarities with the histology of acute GvHD [239]. However, when the clinical situation of patients after allogeneic HSCT is taken into account, none of these diseases represents a true differential diagnosis anymore.

In contrast, there are a number of lesions which, due to their potential occurrence in the posttransplant period and due to their histological resemblance with acute GvHD, pose problems in the differential diagnosis (Table 5.2). These are toxic skin lesions that can be induced by the preparatory chemoradiation conditioning of patients [66, 83, 168, 194, 197, 234, 289, 291], the most severe being Lyell syndrome (toxic epidermal necrolysis).

There also is a considerable overlap in the histomorphology of acute GvHD with drug eruptions of the interface type [3, 227] and with viral infections such as HSV, CMV, and VZV [325]. The similarity in the histological picture primarily results from the occurrence of scattered individual apoptotic keratinocytes and a more or less pronounced lymphocytic infiltration of the upper dermis and lower epidermis [168]. A lymphocytic infiltrate, while necessary for the histological diagnosis of acute GvHD, is also present in most dermatitides, irrespective of etiology, if they last for several weeks [3]. Therefore, this type of inflammatory reaction per se is not a discriminator. And this constitutes the diagnostic dilemma of acute GvHD. The inflammatory infiltrate in most drug eruptions, however, contains neutrophils. Also some of the viral infections may exhibit multinucleated giant cells. Neither of these phenomena occur in acute GvHD. Immunohistology and virological testing may provide further assistance in the differential diagnosis.

Most of the skin lesions important in the differential diagnosis of acute cutaneous GvHD, listed in Table 5.2, are directly or indirectly connected

Table 5.2. Differential diagnosis of acute GvHD of the skin

1. Toxic skin lesions due to pretransplant chemoradiation conditioning
2. Drug eruptions of the interface type, e.g. by GvHD-prophylaxis
3. Viral infections of skin, e.g. by HSV, CMV, VZV
4. Skin lesions due to underlying disease, e.g. in Omenn's syndrome

HSV, herpes simplex virus; CMV, cytomegalovirus; VZV, varicella zoster virus.

with allogeneic HSCT. This implies that patients developing acute GvHD in another clinical context, e. g., after blood transfusion, only rarely exhibit skin lesions that raise problems in the differential diagnosis of GvHD. The exception to this rule are diseases such as Omenn's syndrome, which frequently shows a priori skin involvement (Table 5.2). Basically the skin rash in Omenn's syndrome, a SCID due to partial recombination activating gene (RAG) 1 and 2 deficiency [280], is difficult to distinguish clinically and histologically from cutaneous GvHD after MFT in patients with SCID. However, the clarification of the differential diagnosis is possible by HLA typing: Whereas the T-lymphocytes in infants with SCID and GvHD are of maternal origin, the T-cells in Omenn's syndrome are of patient origin [14]. In addition, the skin changes in infants with that condition lack keratinocyte apoptosis [145].

Three different entities must then be distinguished in infants with SCID and skin rash: (1) MFT-GvHD; (2) TA-GvHD; and (3) cutaneous involvement by Omenn's syndrome.

Finally, when discussing the differential diagnosis of acute GvHD one should point out that in fact there are several types of lesions induced by or associated with GvHD (Table 5.3):

1. Fully established lesions of moderate severity that histomorphologically show the characteristics of acute GvHD.
2. Very early or very mild lesions that histomorphologically are not characteristic of acute GvHD.

Although both types of lesions are induced by GvHD only the former can be recognized and safely diagnosed histologically.

3. In addition there are lesions that are not induced by but may be associated with GvHD. These are tissue changes such as drug eruptions or viral infections which must be distinguished from GvHD (Table 5.3).

Table 5.3. Histomorphological types of lesions occurring in the context of GvHD

---

1. GvHD lesions, histomorphologically characteristic:
   Lymphocytic infiltration of target tissue, apoptosis of individual target cells, moderate severity of lesions, predominantly induced by cytotoxic T-cells?

2. GvHD lesions, histomorphologically not characteristic:
   No lymphocytic infiltration of target tissue[a], apoptosis of individual target cells possible, early or mild lesions, predominantly induced by cytokines?

3. GvHD-associated lesions, histomorphologically variable:
   Mixed cellular infiltration of host tissue, apoptosis or necrosis of cells possible, different severity of lesions, induced by drug toxicity or microbial infections!

---

[a] Not detectable by routine histology.

Insufficient awareness of the existence of these different types of lesions is one reason for the present confusion about the histopathology of acute and chronic GvHD.

5.1.7 Histodiagnostic Aspects of Acute GvHD of the Skin

Sometimes pathologists, including the writer, prefer evaluating biopsies without prior knowledge of the clinical background in order to assure more objective analysis of the lesions. This is a "self-imposed diagnostic discipline, and not a hardship to be imposed by the clinical colleague through withholding clinical information" [79]. While such a purely histomorphological analysis ("blind diagnosis") may be adequate in diseases showing a characteristic histopathology (e.g., benign or malignant tumors), clinical information will greatly assist in the histodiagnostic assessment of less characteristic lesions.

Consider the histomorphological evaluation of inflammatory skin diseases. Here a close clinicopathological correlation is self-evident. Paul Gerson Unna, a long time ago (1928), impressively formulated what is required for a reliable diagnosis: "From the patient to the microscope and back to the patient" [3]. Unfortunately, this is not possible for today's pathologist. Therefore, the clinician is depended on to provide some information on the case history and the gross findings (Table 5.4).

There is another reason why clinical data and a close clinicopathological correlation can improve the accuracy of histological diagnosis. As is evident from Table 5.5, the clinical, histomorphological, and immunohistological assessment of GvHD each have advantages as well as disadvantages. For example, in patients developing GvHD it is difficult to follow the sequence of events at the histological level by biopsy. However, if one takes a look at Table 5.5 it should appear plausible that a combination of the findings obtained by the three different methods can increase the reliability of the GvHD diagnosis.

Table 5.4. Clinical data useful for interpretation of biopsies in the context of GvHD

---

1. Underlying disease of patient?
2. Blood transfusions given to patient?
3. If performed: mode and date of HSCT?
4. Pretransplant conditioning regimen?
5. Blood cell counts of patient?
6. Date and site of biopsy?
7. Questions to be answered by pathologist?

HSCT, hematopoietic stem cell transplantation.

Table 5.5. Advantages and disadvantages of clinical, histomorphological, and immunohistological assessment of GvHD

Assessment	Advantages	Disadvantages
Clinical	Large area of observation Follow up possible	Subjective assessment of most parameters
Histomorphological	Objective assessment of criteria Good reproducibility	Small biopsy, sampling error Momentary picture only
Immunohistological	Assessment of specific features Good reproducibilitiy	Small biopsy, sampling error Momentary picture only

Before performing a skin biopsy the clinician should define a clear question to be answered by the pathologist [94]:

1. Is the biopsy intended primarily to confirm the clinical diagnosis?
2. Should the biopsy distinguish between several diagnostic possibilities?
3. Is the purpose of the biopsy to evaluate efficacy of treatment?

It is obvious that the first and the third question will be much easier to answer than the second question. Still, if the interpretation of biopsies is made in conjunction with adequate clinical information, then it may be possible to answer the second question as well. Involvement, for example, of extracutaneous GvHD target organs such as the liver or GIT can assist in the correct interpretation or evaluation of a skin biopsy not diagnostic on its own.

There are a number of practical aspects that should be taken into consideration when trying to establish a GvHD diagnosis by skin biopsy (Table 5.6). Optimal timing of biopsies is of major importance in particular in patients after allogeneic HSCT. While in the early period (10–25 days) after transplantation conditioning-induced damage of skin frequently interferes with the histological diagnosis of acute GvHD, the discriminatory power of a histomorphological assessment is considerably increased at a later time [180]. Also, since the presence of an inflammatory infiltrate plays a pivotal role in the histological diagnosis of acute GvHD, and since such infiltrates frequently are not yet present immediately after onset of the rash, skin biopsies should not be taken until 24–48 hours later [88, 136].

Similarly, very early or very mild GvHD lesions histologically often show only nonspecific changes that can be easily confused with low-grade drug or

Table 5.6. Guidelines for performing skin biopsies to diagnose acute GvHD

1. Optimal timing of skin biopsy:
   After conditioning effects have subsided
   Not immediately but 24–48 h after onset of the skin rash
   Before starting GvHD therapy
2. Repeated skin biopsies may be required, e.g. in early phase of acute GvHD
3. Serial sections of paraffin-embedded probes may be necessary, e.g. in focal GvHD with predominant follicular involvement
4. Pretransplant base line biopsy useful in patients with skin involvement of underlying disease, e.g., in Omenn's syndrome, Wiskott-Aldrich syndrome

radiation effects [162, 227, 352]. Clearly, repeated skin biopsies are called for to provide information on the sequence of developing pathological events during the manifestation of acute GvHD. In one study of 1,180 biopsies from 368 adult and pediatric patients after allogeneic HSCT, the diagnosis of acute GvHD could be established histologically by one skin biopsy in 64% of cases, by two consecutive skin biopsies in 86%, and by three consecutive skin biopsies in more than 95% [144].

If acute GvHD of skin is fully established, the histological picture "can be recognized at a glance" [277]. However, in early low grade acute GvHD, lesions may be focal, affecting the hair follicles only (Fig. 5.11). Macroscopically such predominant follicular involvement ("follicular GvHD") has a punctate appearance. Serial sections of the corresponding skin biopsy may be required to establish the histological diagnosis (Table 5.6).

A recent reappraisal of the histopathological criteria for the diagnosis of acute GvHD shows a surprising intra- and interobserver reliability in rating cutaneous GvHD [208]. In particular, in established acute GvHD there was a good diagnostic accuracy and perfect agreement among the three participating pathologists [208]. This was not the case for early acute GvHD [352].

Some guidelines for the histological diagnosis of acute GvHD of skin are listed in Table 5.7. The recommendations given are based on the routine histopathological evaluation of skin biopsies from adult and pediatric patients. Overall, a correct diagnosis of acute GvHD can be expected by evaluation of one skin biopsy in about 65% of cases [136]. This agrees well with the published sensitivity of the histodiagnosis of acute GvHD of 67%, a specificity of 78%, and a positive predictive value of 80% [234].

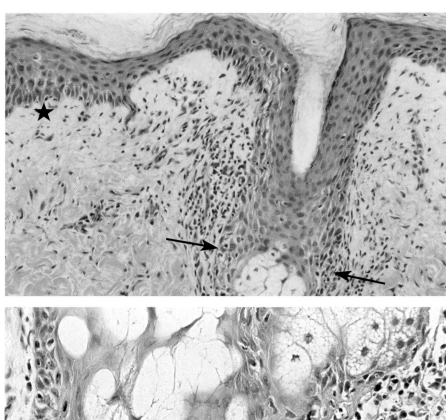

a

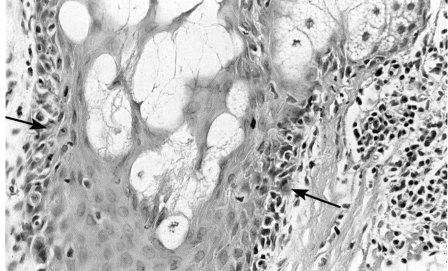

b

Fig. 5.11 a, b. "Follicular GvHD" of the skin. Selective involvement of a hair follicle by acute GvHD. Lymphocytic infiltration of the pilosebaceous unit (*arrows*). Remaining epidermis unremarkable (*asterisk*). Biopsy of a 7-year-old female patient with FA obtained 10 days after HLA-identical unrelated allogeneic BMT. Subsequently the child developed full-blown acute GvHD of the skin and GIT. H&E, **a** ×168, **b** ×328

Table 5.7. Guidelines for histological diagnosis of acute GvHD of the skin

1. GvHD is an immunopathological process characterized by interaction of allo-reactive T-lymphocytes with distinct target tissues. Basically, both components should be demonstrable within GvHD lesions.

2. The predilection sites of acute GvHD of the skin are the rete ridges of the epidermis and the parafollicular bulges. Epithelial stem cells, the targets of acute GvHD, are localized here.

3. Histological criteria of acute cutaneous GvHD are apoptosis of individual keratinocytes and epidermotropic lymphocytic infiltration, concentrated at the dermo-epidermal junction. Both phenomena are crucial for diagnosis.

4. Apoptotic keratinocytes are a necessary but not a sufficient prerequisite for the histological diagnosis of acute GvHD. The same holds true for epidermotropic lymphocytic infiltrates.

5. Low-grade tissue changes, frequently observed in the early phase of acute GvHD, are diagnostically unreliable and possess no discriminatory power.

6. The diagnostic value of biopsies increases with time after allogeneic HSCT and with the number of organs affected by GvHD.

7. A close clinicopathological correlation is of utmost importance for a reliable diagnosis and helps in avoiding diagnostic pitfalls.

HSCT, hematopoietic stem cell transplantation.

5.2 Histological Features of Acute GvHD of the Liver

In about 40% to 60% of patients with acute GvHD the liver participates in the alloimmune process [255]. The hepatic involvement clinically is much less apparent and more difficult to recognize than acute GvHD of the skin. This theoretically would favor the use of liver biopsies for diagnostic clarification. Whereas skin biopsies can be obtained without difficulty and can be repeated on request, liver biopsies, e.g., in patients with thrombocytopenia, are in contrast more risky and cannot be taken at will. Understandably, much less is known of the histopathology of GvHD of the liver than of the skin. Furthermore, the histological diagnosis of acute hepatic GvHD appears to be more difficult than of other GvHD target organs [197].

5.2.1 Early Acute GvHD of the Liver

Initially the liver tissue shows a mild lymphocytic infiltrate within the portal triads accompanied by cytoplasmic vacuolization and nuclear pleomorphism of the epithelia of small bile ducts (Fig. 5.12; [63, 277]). The infiltrates

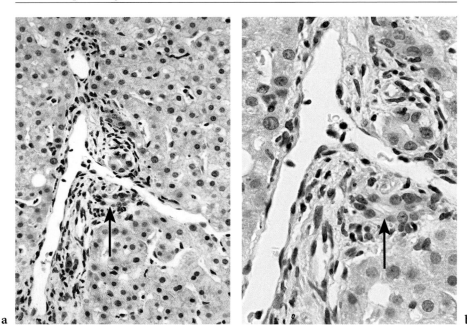

a   b

Fig. 5.12 a, b. Early histopathological changes in acute GvHD of the liver. Slight lymphocytic infiltration of portal triad and small bile ducts (*arrows*). Biopsy of a 5-month-old male infant with SCID obtained 3 months after HLA-nonidentical allogeneic BMT. The child also had low-grade acute GvHD of the skin. H & E, **a** ×210, **b** ×420

may contain single eosinophils but usually no neutrophils or plasma cells. These early hepatic changes are not histologically diagnostic [286, 291]. However, 1–2 weeks after the onset of acute GvHD, clinically evident by the skin rash, a more characteristic histomorphological picture can be observed.

5.2.2 Established Acute GvHD of the Liver

When the hepatic alloreaction progresses, bile duct abnormalities become more pronounced. A distinct lymphocytic infiltration of the portal triads appears, along with atypia, apoptosis, and sloughing of epithelial cells into the bile duct lumen [63]. Cholestasis is observed frequently, while oncocytic metaplasia of bile duct epithelium appears to be a rare event [37]. Although the non-suppurative lymphocytic triaditis may be only mild, dysplastic changes of the small bile ducts are usually prominent (Fig. 5.13). Occasionally, lymphocytic infiltration of and damage to the venous endothelium,

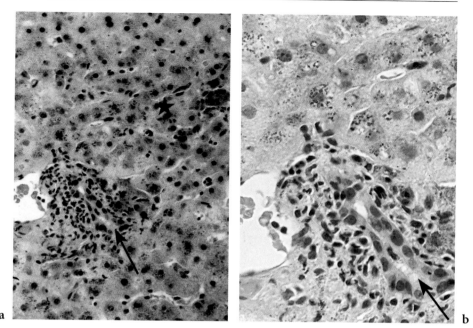

Fig. 5.13 a, b. Established acute GvHD of the liver. Non-suppurative lymphocytic triaditis with distinct nuclear hyperchromasia and pleomorphism of the bile duct epithelium (*arrows*). Focal siderosis of liver tissue (*asterisk*). Biopsy of an 18-year-old female patient with FA obtained 50 days after allogeneic BMT. Acute GvHD of the skin was also present. H&E, a ×210, b ×420

called venular endotheliitis, is present [63, 325]. This is by no means a constant finding, however [9]. Obliterative arteriopathy (obliterative endarteritis), characteristic of liver allograft rejection [249], does not occur in hepatic GvHD [76, 202].

The relative small number of lymphocytes present in acute GvHD of the liver has frustrated many investigators [63, 76, 286, 329]. As previously outlined in detail, this most likely is due to pretransplant cytoreductive conditioning and posttransplant immunosuppression [76, 286]. Diagnostically more important is the finding that in acute hepatic GvHD after allogeneic HSCT the majority of lymphocytes infiltrating the portal triads and bile ducts are of the donor genotype [9]. This indicates that the lesions observed in fact represent the manifestation of an alloreaction in the liver [269, 275, 276].

5.2.3 Severity of Acute GvHD of the Liver

The severity of hepatic involvement in acute GvHD varies from slight to very strong. In the latter case the progressive destruction of small bile ducts may result in a so-called "vanishing bile duct syndrome" [63]. Lerner et al. [197] have devised a histological grading system, exclusively based on the extent of lesions (epithelial damage and destruction) of small bile ducts:

Grade I: <25%
Grade II: 25%–49%
Grade III: 50%–74%
Grade IV: ≥75%

The results of this scoring is included in the overall histological grading of acute GvHD (see Table 5.10).

5.2.4 Time Course of Acute GvHD of the Liver

In contrast to acute GvHD of the skin there are only few histomorphological studies on the time course of acute GvHD of the liver employing sequential biopsies [286]. Nevertheless, from these studies it is evident that biopsies taken at a later time, that is beyond 3 months after transplantation, more frequently show bile duct dropout and portal fibrosis than do those taken earlier. This indicates that progression of acute GvHD results in increasing bile duct destruction. Early diagnosis and treatment are obviously important. Yet for reasons outlined before, liver biopsies are performed in the patients discussed here only rarely.

In this context one should point out that the terms "acute" or "chronic" hepatic GvHD relate more to the time of onset of the disease than to distinct histological features [277, 278]. In other words, the histomorphology of acute and chronic GvHD of the liver shows a gradual transition and no clear-cut differences.

There is another important point to be made concerning the time course of hepatic GvHD. Figure 5.14 illustrates the result of skin and liver follow-up biopsies in a patient with reticular dysgenesis (RD) developing acute GvHD after allogeneic BMT. As is evident from the data shown in the figure, the cutaneous GvHD after treatment with prednisolone and CSA disappeared whereas the hepatic GvHD persisted. This different response of GvHD lesions in different target organs to immunosuppressive therapy is by no means unusual but rather common. It is evident that such observations have important implications.

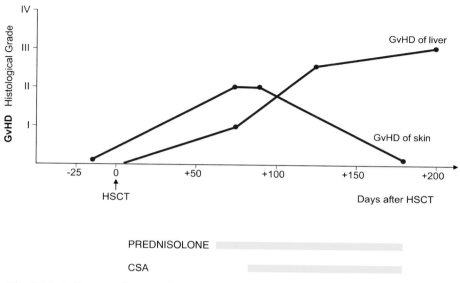

Fig. 5.14. Influence of GvHD therapy on the course of GvHD of the liver and skin as determined by follow-up biopsies (•) in a male infant with RD after HLA-nonidentical related allogeneic BMT. Transplantation was performed $2^{1}/_{2}$ months after birth without conditioning and without GvHD prophylaxis. The first skin biopsy was taken 15 days before BMT. Note the different course of hepatic and cutaneous GvHD. CSA, cyclosporine A; RD, reticular dysgenesis

5.2.5 Histological Criteria of Acute GvHD of the Liver

Most pathologists agree that pathological changes of the small interlobular bile ducts are a conditio sine qua non for the histological diagnosis of hepatic GvHD [76]. Dysplasia and destruction of bile duct epithelia associated with portal lymphocytic infiltration are the most consistent and the most characteristic findings [9, 63, 325]. Nevertheless, these lesions are not pathognomonic and only in conjunction with the clinical context permit the diagnosis of hepatic GvHD [291]. Since recognition of apoptosis in bile duct epithelium is much more difficult than in the epidermis, this change does not represent a histological criterion for the diagnosis of acute hepatic GvHD.

5.2.6 Differential Diagnosis of Acute GvHD of the Liver

First of all, it is important to point out that the liver tissue of patients with diseases such as leukemia or other malignancies frequently shows hepatic damage independent of GvHD as a result of cytostatic chemotherapy, pre-

Table 5.8. Differential diagnosis of acute GvHD of the liver

1. Toxic hepatic damage including VOD due to pretransplant cytoablative chemotherapy
2. Drug-induced hepatopathia, e. g., by GvHD prophylaxis
3. Viral infections of liver, e. g., by HCV, CMV, HSV

VOD, venoocclusive disease; HCV, hepatitis C virus; CMV, cytomegalovirus; HSV, herpes simplex virus.

transplant conditioning, and/or posttransplant GvHD prophylaxis. Included are individual hepatocyte necroses (Councilman bodies), fatty change of liver parenchyma, siderosis, and assorted mesenchymal reactions [291, 325]. Such tissue alterations are commonly seen histologically in addition to the lesions induced by GvHD. Pretransplant irradiation, unlike the effects seen in skin and gut, does not induce liver damage and therefore does not interfere with the diagnosis of acute hepatic GvHD [291].

In contrast, there is some overlap of the histomorphology of acute hepatic GvHD and of several other diseases involving the liver. This holds true for drug-induced hepatic damage including veno-occlusive disease (VOD), for viral infections such as hepatitis C virus (HCV), cytomegalovirus (CMV), herpes simplex virus (HSV), and, rarely, for hepatic infections by bacteria or fungi. A list of major complications that play a role in the clinical and histological differential diagnosis of acute hepatic GvHD is given in Table 5.8.

While some authors assume that a distinction between GvHD and most of the liver lesions listed in the table is possible histomorphologically [202, 277, 325] other authors do not [87]. All agree that the histological evaluation of liver biopsies after allogeneic HSCT gets more informative and reliable as time passes postoperatively [63, 325]. In addition, some of the infectious agents mentioned in Table 5.8 can be specifically identified by immunohistology or virology [60].

5.2.7 Histodiagnostic Aspects of Acute GvHD of the Liver

While liver biopsies are an important diagnostic tool for chronic GvHD, they are not widely used for the diagnosis of acute hepatic GvHD [63]. This is due to several reasons:

1. In most patients hepatic GvHD is associated with or follows acute GvHD of other organs, in particular of skin [325]. Therefore, when a patient with histologically proved skin GvHD develops clinical symptoms compatible with hepatic GvHD a liver biopsy is not necessary for reliable diagnosis [329].

2. In the early phase of acute GvHD, that is, up to 35 days after transplantation, liver biopsies often do not yet show characteristic lesions. Diagnostically relevant pathological changes of the bile ducts are more frequently present following that interval [286].
3. Because of the patchy distribution of lesions, a needle biopsy may give a false-negative result [63].
4. Finally, as already mentioned, a liver biopsy may be risky in patients with thrombocytopenia.

Overall, the histological diagnosis of acute GvHD of the liver does have a sensitivity of 66 %, a specificity of 91 % and a predictive value of 86 % [286].

5.3 Histological Features of Acute GvHD of the Gastrointestinal Tract

The GIT is affected by acute GvHD in about 30 %–50 % of recipients of allogeneic BMT [56, 342]. All parts of the GIT can be affected, but a number of studies indicate that lesions are most marked in the ileum and colon and that damage of the stomach, duodenum, jejunum, and rectum is less severe [112, 273, 289]. In most instances acute gastrointestinal GvHD develops simultaneously with or shortly after GvHD of the skin. Isolated manifestation of GvHD in the GIT is uncommon [86].

Acute intestinal disease plays an important pathophysiological role in the amplification of systemic GvHD and profoundly influences the prognosis of patients [86, 146]. Severe GvHD of the gut is in fact the most frequent cause of death from acute GvHD [56, 277].

5.3.1 Early Acute GvHD of the Gastrointestinal Tract

Acute GvHD of the gut starts with a focal increase in the number of lymphocytes within the lamina propria, edema, and "granular necrosis" of individual epithelial cells in the crypts of the intestinal mucosa [247, 273, 293, 329]. "Granular necrosis" of enterocytes actually represents apoptotic cell death [293, 311]. Microscopically, the phenomenon is characterized by an intraepithelial vacuole filled with karyorrhectic debris (Fig. 5.15). The apoptotic bodies most likely are derived from proliferating epithelial stem cells that are the targets for acute GvHD in the gut [269]. Since many patients in the first weeks after allogeneic HSCT have a profound leukopenia, in general there is only a scant inflammatory infiltrate [293]. Overall, early intestinal GvHD lesions are histomorphologically nonspecific and nondiagnostic.

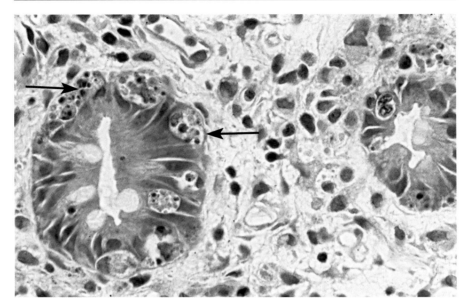

Fig. 5.15. Early acute GvHD of the colon. Sparse infiltration of the lamina propria by lymphocytes and single eosinophils. Multiple apoptotic crypt cells (*arrows*). Biopsy of a 9 year-old male patient with ALL obtained 19 days after HLA-identical allogeneic BMT. Acute GvHD of the skin was also present. H & E, × 672

Early acute GvHD of the stomach, due to lack of "physiological inflammation," can be identified more easily. Here, apoptotic cell death primarily occurs in the neck region of the gastric mucosa [277, 293].

5.3.2 Established Acute GvHD of the Gastrointestinal Tract

Lesions show more characteristic histological features as the alloreaction progresses. Crypts appear that exhibit numerous apoptotic bodies and much cellular debris in the dilated lumen. Because of their distinct appearance (Fig. 5.16) these lesions have been termed "exploding crypts" by Sale et al. [273]. Although they are not pathognomonic for acute GvHD, "exploding crypts" represent a very characteristic finding [273, 277, 325]. Fully developed GvHD lesions of the gut also show increased numbers of intraepithelial lymphocytes [311].

During the further course of disease the "exploding crypt" is often transformed into a histologically less characteristic lesion, a "crypt abscess" [273, 277]. This is defined as a crypt containing cellular debris and numerous polymorphonuclear leukocytes in the dilated lumen (Fig. 5.17 [273]). "Crypt

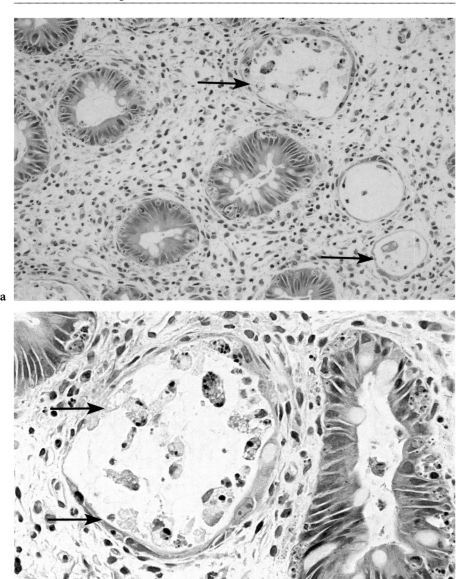

Fig. 5.16a, b. Established acute GvHD of the colon. Moderate lymphocytic infiltration of the lamina propria. Several typical "exploding crypts" (*arrows*). Biopsy of the same patient as in Fig. 5.15, but obtained 26 days after BMT. H & E, **a** × 210, **b** × 420

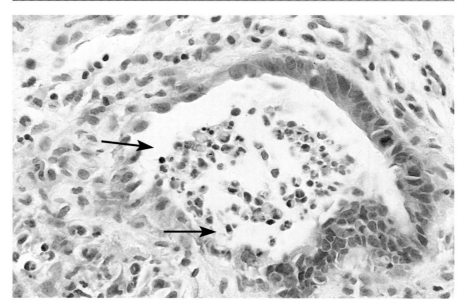

Fig. 5.17. Acute GvHD of the colon. "Crypt abscess" (*arrows*) with polymorpho-nuclear leukocytes and cellular debris within the crypt lumen. Sparse lymphocytic infiltration of the lamina propria. Biopsy of a 5 year-old male patient with MHC class II-deficiency obtained 82 days after HLA-nonidentical allogeneic BMT. Acute GvHD of the skin was also present. H & E, × 420

abscesses" are not specific for GvHD but also occur in ulcerative colitis and other diseases of the gut. If intestinal GvHD progresses the result may be crypt dropout, focal or diffuse mucosal ulceration, and denudation (Fig. 5.18 [247, 298, 342]).

Fully developed acute GvHD lesions in the stomach differ somewhat from the histopathological findings in the gut. Here, in most instances, the lesions are less severe and are primarily characterized by lymphocytic inflammation and apoptosis. These findings apply to the gastric corpus (Fig. 5.19) as well as the antrum (Fig. 5.20). In contrast to nonspecific superficial lymphocytic gastritis the lymphocytic infiltration of the stomach in acute GvHD has a tendency to spread from the basis of the mucosa to the surface.

The histomorphological picture of acute GvHD of the duodenum closely resembles disease manifestations in the other sections of the gut (Fig. 5.21).

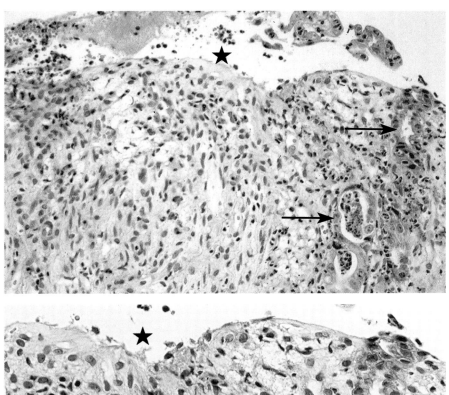

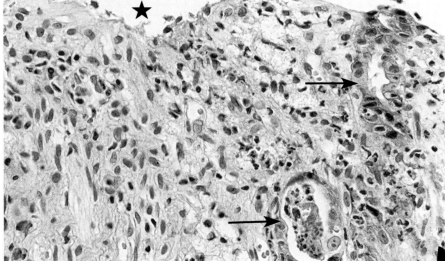

Fig. 5.18a, b. Acute GvHD of the colon. Extensive mucosal ulceration with denuda-tion (*asterisks*). At higher magnification some crypt residues are visible (*arrows*). Biopsy of a 38-year-old male patient with CML obtained 65 days after allogeneic BMT. Acute GvHD of the skin was present also. H&E, **a** ×210, **b** ×420

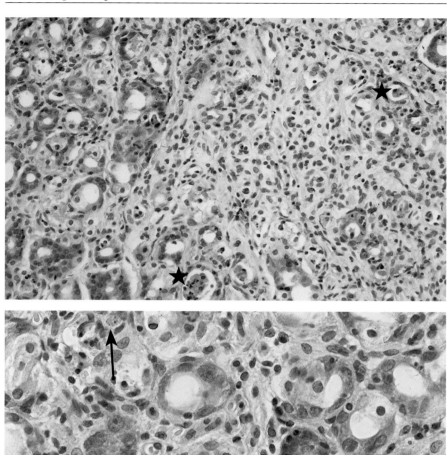

Fig. 5.19a, b. Acute GvHD of the gastric corpus. Slight irregularity of glands and sparse lymphocytic infiltration. Cellular debris in the lumen of single glands (*asterisks*) and rare apoptotic bodies (*arrow*). Biopsy of a 21-year-old male patient with acute undifferentiated leukemia (AUL) obtained 28 days after HLA-identical allogeneic BMT. Marked acute GvHD of the skin and liver was also present. H & E, **a** ×210, **b** ×420

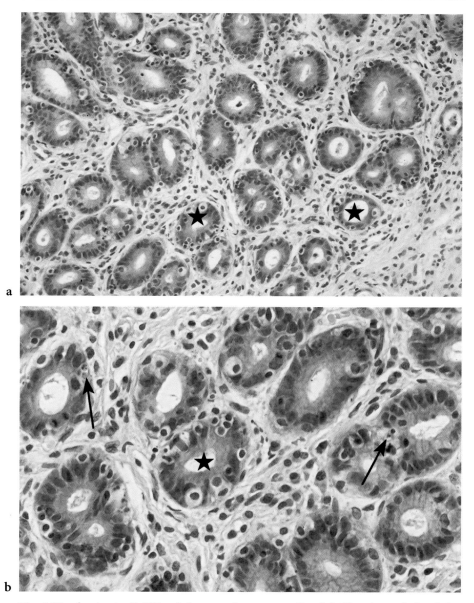

Fig. 5.20a, b. Acute GvHD of the gastric antrum. Focal infiltration of glandular epithelium by lymphocytes (*asterisks*). Single apoptotic bodies present (*arrows*). The lamina propria also contains some plasma cells. Biopsy of the same patient as in Fig. 5.19. H & E, **a** × 210, **b** × 420

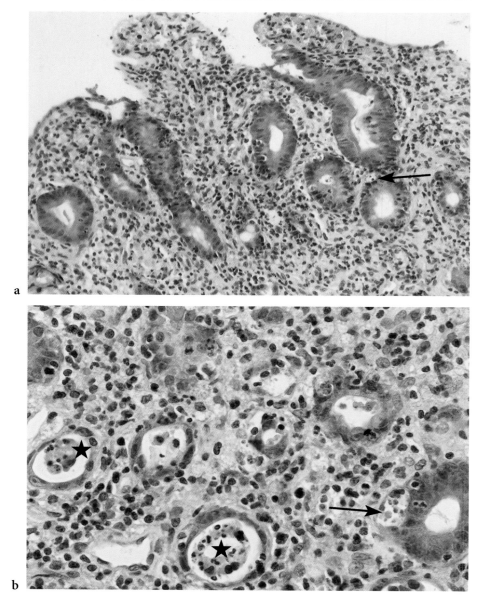

Fig. 5.21 a, b. Acute GvHD of the duodenum. Increased infiltration of the mucosa by lymphocytes and other mononuclear cells. Several apoptotic bodies (*arrows*) and "exploding crypts" (*asterisks*). Biopsy of the same patient as in Fig. 5.19. H&E, **a** × 210, **b** × 420

5.3.3 Severity of Acute GvHD of the Gastrointestinal Tract

The involvement of the GIT varies from patient to patient, from focal to diffuse, and from limited to extensive. These differences in the severity and extent of lesions are the basis for the histological grading of acute gastrointestinal GvHD [197]:

Grade I: Single cell apoptosis of crypt or gland epithelium
Grade II: Destruction of single crypts or glands
Grade III: Focal mucosal ulceration
Grade IV: Diffuse mucosal ulceration with denudation

The results of this scoring are used for the overall histological grading of acute GvHD (see Table 5.10). As mentioned before, the various parts of the GIT are affected by acute GvHD to a different extent, the most severe lesions being found in the ileum and colon. In contrast, lesions in the upper GIT, in particular in the stomach, are usually less severe.

5.3.4 Time Course of Acute GvHD of the Gastrointestinal Tract

The onset, severity, and course of acute GvHD of the GIT basically depends on the same factors influencing acute GvHD of the skin and liver. However, in contrast to the latter organs, the presence of large numbers of microorganisms in the lower intestinal tract represents an additional pathogenetic factor influencing the course and outcome [277]. If one takes into account the potential complications of severe gastrointestinal GvHD (e.g., hemorrhage, infection, sepsis) it is not surprising that patients with acute GvHD of the gut have a high mortality of 30%–60% [56].

Though usually not as seriously damaged as other sections of the gut, studies of consecutive rectal biopsies still have been found to show a good correlation with the clinical course of acute GvHD of the gastrointestinal tract [273].

5.3.5 Histological Criteria of Acute GvHD of the Gastrointestinal Tract

Early GvHD of the GIT histologically exhibits uncharacteristic changes such as edema, sparse lymphocytic infiltration, and single apoptotic bodies. Since apoptosis occurs physiologically in the gastrointestinal mucosa [137] and since it may increase considerably after chemoradiation conditioning, low-grade changes (grade I) with single apoptotic bodies in the first 20–30 days after allogeneic HSCT are nondiagnostic [291, 293, 298]. In contrast, a reliable diagnosis is possible if lesions show "exploding crypts" (grade II), the histological hallmark of acute GvHD of the gut [273, 277]. As before, although "exploding crypts" are very characteristic of GvHD, they are not pathognomonic.

"Crypt abscesses," because of their nonspecific nature, do not represent a safe histomorphological criterion. Nor does mucosal ulceration, which may occur in severe forms of gastrointestinal GvHD (grade III–IV), but also in many other destructive processes of the GIT [271]. In short, very mild and very severe pathological changes are diagnostically equivocal.

5.3.6 Differential Diagnosis of Acute GvHD of the Gastrointestinal Tract

First, one should distinguish the gastrointestinal diseases that are *clinically* similar to acute GvHD, and have to be taken into consideration because they may occur in patients at risk of developing GvHD, from those that are *histomorphologically* similar and also require such consideration. With respect to the former group, one should mention diseases such as ulcerative colitis, ischemic colitis, intestinal vasculitis, and Crohn's disease [187].

Gastrointestinal diseases belonging to the latter group are listed in Table 5.9. Most important in mimicking acute GvHD of GIT are lesions caused by bone marrow-ablative chemotherapy and/or total body irradiation [339] observed within the first 20–30 days after transplantation. Lesions histologically resembling GvHD may also be induced by drugs (e. g., those used for GvHD prophylaxis), by viral infections (e. g., CMV, HSV) and, occasionally, by bacterial or fungal infections of the gut [49, 86, 277, 291, 293, 298, 325, 329, 339]. Although there is a considerable overlap of histomorphological patterns, these lesions can often be distinguished from acute GvHD by repeated biopsies, microbial studies, and/or careful clinicopathological correlation.

Sometimes gastrointestinal GvHD and opportunistic infections [212, 270] occur simultaneously. In these cases a particularly careful diagnostic work-up is required. Although many of the opportunistic infections can be recognized by histomorphology or immunohistology [22, 106, 221], a detailed microbiological analysis is also needed.

Thanks to the absence of chemoradiation conditioning effects, there are much fewer problems of differential diagnosis in TA-GvHD of GIT.

Table 5.9. Differential diagnosis of acute GvHD of the gastrointestinal tract

1. Toxic gastrointestinal lesions due to pretransplant conditioning
2. Drug-induced gastrointestinal lesions, e. g., by GvHD prophylaxis
3. Viral infections of the gastrointestinal tract, e. g., by CMV, HSV
4. Bacterial or fungal infections of the gastrointestinal tract

CMV, cytomegalovirus; HSV, herpes simplex virus.

5.3.7 Histodiagnostic Aspects of Acute GvHD of the Gastrointestinal Tract

Mucosal biopsies play a significant role in the histomorphological diagnosis of acute GvHD of the GIT. However, this is true only after the disappearance of the chemoradiation damage which mimics acute GvHD. Timing of gastrointestinal biopsies is then of great importance. Within the first 20 – 30 days after allogeneic HSCT the histodiagnosis of acute gastrointestinal GvHD is relatively unreliable [291, 311]. Thereafter biopsy yields increasingly reliable diagnosis [187, 311].

Yet early diagnosis of acute GvHD of the GIT is extremely desirable because of the profound prognostic significance of the gastrointestinal involvement. A major difficulty hinders early diagnosis. In the early phase of the disease GvHD lesions histomorphologically are not characteristic. At this stage lesions cannot be distinguished from those induced by myeloablative pretreatment of patients [291]. In these circumstances the clinicopathological correlation is of utmost importance and can help to avoid misinterpretation of biopsies. If, for instance, the histology of the gastrointestinal lesions is not diagnostic of GvHD, the simultaneous presence of acute GvHD of skin and/or liver will facilitate interpretation of the biopsy.

Rectal, gastric, and duodenal biopsies can all be very useful in GvHD diagnosis [70, 277, 342]. The optimal site for biopsy depends on the clinical symptoms. When diarrhea is present rectal biopsies are in order; when nausea, vomiting, and/or pain of the upper abdomen is present gastroduodenal biopsies are useful [293]. Simultaneous upper and lower endoscopic biopsies have been reported to show a discordance in the diagnosis of GvHD in 28% of patients [261].

Another aspect of the histodiagnosis of gastrointestinal GvHD has come to light from the observation that rectal biopsies in infants with SCID – for unknown reasons – may show GvHD-like histological changes prior to allogeneic HSCT [294, 295, 338]. This renders interpretation of biopsies after HSCT more difficult. In such a situation it is advisable to take a so-called base-line biopsy from the respective infants before starting treatment.

Because of the focal nature of early GvHD lesions, serial sections of gastrointestinal biopsies frequently are useful [311]. Although "blind" histological diagnosis of acute GvHD in gastric biopsies has been possible with a specificity of 76%, a sensitivity of 82%, and a predictive value of 69% [339], the histological evaluation of sections should always be made in conjunction with clinical findings.

5.4 Histological Features of Acute GvHD of Other Organs

Each of the three classic GvHD target organs (skin, liver, GIT) thus far described possesses a prominent epithelial component; the damage induced by GvHD concentrates on this layer where it is relatively easy to identify histomorphologically. What is the situation in non-epithelial organs?

There are a number of other organs and tissues thought to be attacked by acute GvHD. While most authors agree that the bone marrow and the immune system are two such tissues, controversies exist concerning the possible involvement elsewhere. These disputes are due in large part to differences between clinical observations and histomorphological findings. Clinically, many tissue changes developing after allogeneic HSCT are attributed to GvHD whereas histologically, if a characteristic morphologic substrate is lacking, they are not.

This is not surprising if one takes into account that in most of the patients discussed here different pathomechanisms are active, such as GvHD, drug or radiation toxicity, and infection [271]. As a matter of fact, in some of these patients different pathogenetic factors may cooperate to produce one lesion or may act separately to produce several different lesions at the same time [270].

In the present monograph on the clinical and diagnostic pathology of GvHD only such lesions are discussed that have been proven to represent GvHD. Therefore other HSCT-associated complications such as toxic lesions or infections are excluded from this text.

5.4.1 Acute GvHD of the Bone Marrow

Normally the bone marrow in allogeneic HSCT is not a target for acute GvHD. This is because both the bone marrow and the T-cells are derived from the same individual, the donor [133]. However, there are several clinical settings in which the bone marrow may be damaged by acute GvHD, for instance in TA-GvHD, in GvHD in children with SCID, and in GvHD associated with donor lymphocyte infusion (DLI) [138, 182, 266].

In patients with TA-GvHD bone marrow failure with pancytopenia is a frequent and characteristic finding [10]. This is due to the fact that in this setting the bone marrow and the T-cells are derived from two genetical different individuals and that HSCs are particularly sensitive to alloreactive T-cells [133]. The damage induced by acute GvHD finally results in bone marrow hypoplasia or aplasia. Remarkably, TA-GvHD does not occur only in patients with immunodeficiency but – under certain conditions – can also manifest itself in immunocompetent individuals (see p. 9). The clinical course and outcome (mostly lethal) in immunocompetent patients is not different from that in immunocompromised hosts [10].

A second example for damage of the bone marrow by acute GvHD are infants with SCID receiving allogeneic HSCT without pretransplant conditioning. In this situation the marrow may be damaged by acute GvHD resulting in bone marrow hypoplasia or aplasia [265].

Finally, GvHD-associated marrow aplasia is commonly observed in patients with CML and a hematological relapse after HSCT receiving treatment with allogeneic DLI.

It should be noted that acute GvHD of the bone marrow, caused by a classic alloreaction, must be distinguished from non-take, primary graft failure, and graft rejection [223]. None of the latter exhibit specific histomorphological findings.

5.4.2 Acute GvHD of the Lymphatic Organs

It has long been known that lymphatic organs such as the thymus, the lymph nodes, and the spleen can be a target for acute GvHD [325]. Damage to the thymus by acute GvHD is thought to play a prominent role in the induction of the multiorgan syndrome that characterizes chronic GvHD [219]. An intact thymus has been demonstrated to be of fundamental importance for immunological reconstitution in SCID [218].

There are several reports on the histomorphology of acute GvHD in various lymphatic organs [266]. It is frequently difficult to decide whether the lesions observed are in fact caused by GvHD or by some other pathomechanisms also active in many of the patients discussed here [142, 347].

Basically, the histomorphological hallmark of acute GvHD of lymph nodes and other lymphatic organs is a profound depletion of lymphocytes (Fig. 5.22). In the long run the process results in a more or less complete atrophy of lymphatic tissues, the clinical effect of which is a severe immundeficiency [19, 255]. The histopathology of acute GvHD of the lymphatic organs is generally less characteristic and more poorly defined than that of the three classic target organs.

5.4.3 Acute GvHD of the Lung

There still is no general agreement whether the lung is a target of acute GvHD [203]. While many pathologists cannot identify a characteristic histomorphological substrate [203, 277, 292, 300], most clinicians are convinced that acute GvHD of the lung exists and has a significant prognostic role [7, 70]. The latter assumption is not surprising since pulmonary complications after allogeneic BMT occur in 40%–60% of patients and contribute significantly to morbidity and mortality [203]. However, many of these pulmonary complications are caused by infectious agents or chemoradiation toxicity

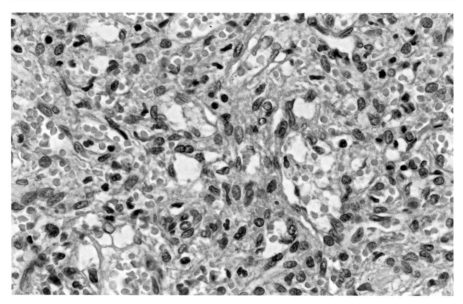

Fig. 5.22. Spleen of a patient with severe acute GvHD. Subtotal lymphocytic depletion of parenchyma. Prominent sinusoids filled with erythrocytes. Post mortem finding in a 15-year-old female patient with AA 45 days after HLA-identical allogeneic BMT. At the time of autopsy acute GvHD was found in the skin, liver, and GIT. H&E, ×420

[19, 22]. The clinicopathological controversy described thus resides in the difficulty of distinguishing between GvHD-induced and GvHD-associated lesions (see Table 5.3).

Tissue changes such as lymphocytic bronchitis and alveolitis are also thought by some authors to represent the histomorphological correlate of an alloreaction of the lung [7, 351]. From the point of view of pathology such lesions are nonspecific and have not been proven to represent pulmonary GvHD [203, 277, 278].

5.5 Histological Grading of Acute GvHD

As previously described, there are several scoring systems for the clinical grading of acute GvHD. By applying these systems an assessment of the severity of acute GvHD and a prediction of the outcome is possible. Since the clinical parameters used are nonspecific per se, a definite GvHD diagnosis must be established by other means. The clinical diagnosis should be confirmed and supplemented by histology [19, 70]. Such a cooperative

Table 5.10. Histological grading of acute GvHD (modified from Lerner et al. [197]; Atkinson [19])

Organ	Grade	Histological criteria
Skin	I	Vacuolar degeneration of basal and suprabasal epidermal cells
	II	Spongiosis and scattered apoptosis of individual keratinocytes
	III	Focal dermo-epidermal separation and cleft formation
	IV	Extensive necrosis of epidermis with denudation
Liver	I	<25% of small bile ducts showing epithelial damage
	II	25%–49% of small bile ducts involved
	III	50%–74% of small bile ducts involved
	IV	75% or more of small bile ducts involved
GIT	I	Single cell apoptosis of crypt or gland epithelium
	II	Destruction of single crypts or glands
	III	Focal mucosal necrosis with ulceration
	IV	Diffuse mucosal necrosis with denudation

GIT, gastrointestinal tract.

effort makes possible a histological grading of the severity of acute GvHD (Table 5.10).

As is evident from Table 5.10, lymphocytic infiltration of lesions does not belong to the criteria of the Lerner rating. This is remarkable since a lymphocytic infiltrate of the epidermis must be present for the histological diagnosis of acute GvHD to be made [88, 154, 208, 234]. A number of authors have proposed that the Lerner grading system should be revised by including lymphocytic infiltration as an additional criterion of acute GvHD grade II.

All grading systems, histological as well as clinical, have advantages and disadvantages. No single one is ideal. The fact that the Lerner grading system (Table 5.10) is reproducible [208], has a high predictive value [19], and has been widely employed for more than 25 years indicates that it is useful and reliable.

6 Histopathological Manifestations of Chronic GvHD

Chronic GvHD develops in about 30%–50% of patients after related donor BMT [16]. In addition to the three classic targets of acute GvHD – skin, liver, and GIT – it may involve many other organs and tissues [176, 255, 278, 284]. Chronic GvHD can manifest early or late, in a localized or generalized way, and, according to the type of onset, as progressive, quiescent, or de novo disease. In view of so many clinical variables it is not surprising that the histopathology of chronic GvHD also differs considerably. The organ most frequently affected is the skin.

6.1 Histological Features of Chronic GvHD of the Skin

The skin is involved in 80%–90% of patients with chronic GvHD [77, 176, 253]. The cutaneous lesions develop either as a continuation of acute GvHD (progressive type), after a latent period (quiescent type), or without prior acute GvHD (de novo type).

Histomorphologically two variants can be distinguished: lichenoid lesions occurring in the early phase and sclerodermatous (sclerodermoid, sclerotic) lesions occurring in the late phase of the disease [15, 176, 219, 284, 291].

6.1.1 Lichenoid Chronic GvHD

Lichenoid lesions commonly manifest early (3–4 months after HSCT) in the course of chronic cutaneous GvHD, although they have been observed to appear across a wide time range of 33–832 days after BMT [158].

Histomorphologically, lichenoid lesions show slight epidermal hyperplasia and a bandlike lymphocytic infiltration of the upper dermis (Fig. 6.1), close to the dermo-epidermal junction, frequently involving pilar and eccrine units [120, 285]. The inflammatory infiltrate may also contain plasma cells, macrophages, and single eosinophils; it may progress into deep dermal structures or even subcutaneous fat tissue [277]. The infiltrate can focally invade the epidermis as well [95]. Occasionally, individual apoptotic keratinocytes and satellitosis are seen. As a result of basal-cell-layer injury the papillary dermis frequently contains melanophages. Altogether the changes bear a striking resemblance to lichen planus [149].

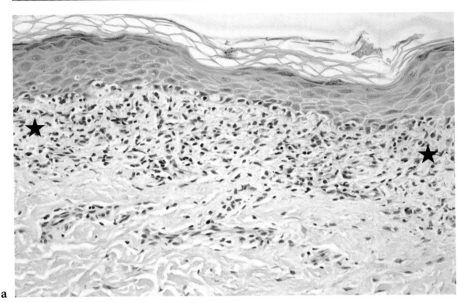

a

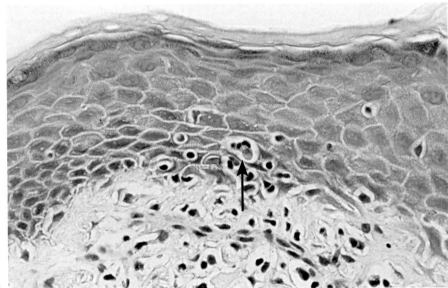

b

Fig. 6.1 a, b. Chronic GvHD of the skin, lichenoid type. Bandlike lymphocytic infiltrate in the upper dermis (*asterisks*). Complete loss of the rete ridges. Single apoptotic keratinocytes with satellitosis (*arrow*). Biopsy of a $7^1/_2$-month-old male infant with SCID obtained 7 months after allogeneic BMT. H & E, **a** ×210, **b** ×420

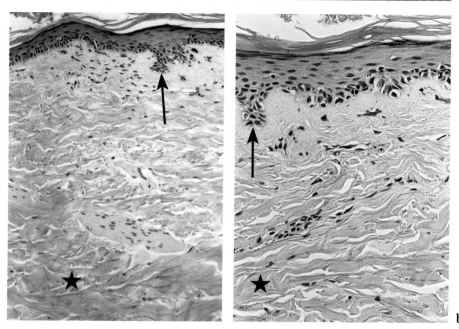

a   b

Fig. 6.2 a, b. Chronic GvHD of the skin, sclerodermatous type. Atrophy of the epidermis with sparse residues of the rete ridges (*arrows*). Deposition of collagen in the reticular dermis (*asterisks*) and atrophy of the adnexae. No inflammatory infiltration. Biopsy of a 10-year-old male patient with AML obtained 2 years after HLA-identical allogeneic BMT. H & E, **a** × 120, **b** × 240

6.1.2 Sclerodermatous Chronic GvHD

In the late phase (6–12 months after HSCT) of chronic cutaneous GvHD a deposition of collagen begins at the interface of the reticular dermis and subcutis. Initially there still may be single sparse perivascular lymphoplasmacytic infiltrates in the dermis. However, with increasing deposition of collagen the changes acquire a scleroderma-like picture (Fig. 6.2). The overlying epidermis most often becomes diffusely atrophic and the rete ridges disappear. There also is atrophy and fibrosis of adnexal structures [120]. Thus, in contrast to acute GvHD, involvement of the eccrine glands is a characteristic of chronic GvHD [219]. The sclerosis of skin may even advance into the subcutaneous fat tissue.

If sclerodermatous GvHD passes through a phase of activity and progression this is evident histologically by inflammation and epidermal single cell apoptosis.

6.1.3 Severity of Chronic GvHD of the Skin

Microscopically as well as grossly there are considerable differences in the severity of tissue changes induced by chronic GvHD. Assessment of the severity of chronic cutaneous GvHD would be meaningful if it would reflect the involvement of internal organs and the prognosis of patients [5]. Treatment with CSA or corticosteroids can significantly modify the histomorphology of lesions, quantitatively as well as qualitatively, and thereby increase the difficulty of such an assessment [176, 335]. Also, the clinical extent of lesions may in fact be more important than the histological severity grade. Chronic GvHD of the generalized type carries a much less favorable prognosis than does the localized type [176]. Assessment of the extent of skin involvement obviously plays a significant prognostic role (see Table 4.3).

6.1.4 Time Course of Chronic GvHD of the Skin

The course of chronic GvHD of the skin over time depends on many different factors. The peak incidence is 1–2 years after transplantation. By 4–5 years the disease usually has resolved, although some cases have lasted for more than 12 years [19].

While the localized type of chronic GvHD in most instances shows nodular induration and dyspigmentation of skin only, the generalized type frequently exhibits severe poikiloderma with diffuse sclerosis, eventually contractures, alopecia, damage or loss of nails, and skin ulcerations [285]. Today, such severe and progressive forms of chronic cutaneous GvHD are rare and, if they occur, they can be slowed down by CSA, corticosteroids, or other measures [335]. It is evident that GvHD prophylaxis and treatment can modify the clinical manifestation as well as the histomorphology of chronic GvHD.

6.1.5 Differential Diagnosis of Chronic GvHD of the Skin

There are a number of skin lesions that resemble chronic cutaneous GvHD histomorphologically. With respect to the lichenoid variant this holds true for lichen ruber planus, lichen planus-like drug eruptions, lichen sclerosus et atrophicus and, occasionally, lupus erythematosus discoides [149, 277, 284]. As far as the sclerodermatous variant is concerned, progressive systemic sclerosis, localized scleroderma, and, rarely, radiation fibrosis have to be considered in the differential diagnosis.

When the clinical setting of patients is taken into consideration, most of the skin lesions mentioned do not represent a true alternative, however, because their occurrence in the given setting is highly unlikely or because they can be excluded clinically. In practice, histomorphologically only lichen

Table 6.1. Differential diagnosis of chronic GvHD of the skin

1. Lichen planus-like drug eruptions
2. Radiation fibrosis of skin
3. Progressive systemic sclerosis

planus-like drug eruptions, radiation fibrosis and, occasionally, progressive systemic sclerosis play a role in the differential diagnosis (Table 6.1).

6.1.6 Histodiagnostic Criteria of Chronic GvHD of the Skin

Since the skin is affected in 80%–90% of patients with chronic GvHD and since 65% of patients have involvement of more than one organ system [253], skin biopsies possess a considerable diagnostic and prognostic potential. Even as a screening test for chronic GvHD skin biopsies have a sensitivity of 68% and a predictive value of 91% [277].

The chief criterion for the histological diagnosis of chronic GvHD of the lichenoid type is a bandlike lymphoplasmacytic infiltrate in the upper dermis that may advance into deep dermal structures and adnexae, and superficially into the basal parts of the overlying epidermis. Sometimes histopathological features characteristic of acute GvHD (e.g., apoptotic bodies, satellitosis) are present as an indication of activity and progression of the disease. The epidermis of lesional skin often is hyperplastic.

Criteria for the histological diagnosis of chronic GvHD of the sclerodermatous type are sclerosis of the dermis with homogenization of collagen bundles, atrophy of the epidermis, disappearance of the rete ridges, and atrophy of the skin adnexae. Sometimes the dermis contains sparse perivascular lymphocytic infiltrates.

6.2 Histological Features of Chronic GvHD of the Liver

The liver is involved in about 30% of patients with chronic GvHD [253]. There are several peculiarities of chronic hepatic GvHD. Most authors agree that liver biopsies possess considerable diagnostic value [63, 76, 255, 277]. As a matter of fact, the diagnosis of chronic GvHD of the liver rests on three parameters: persistent elevation of alkaline phosphatase levels in blood, clinical involvement of other organs by chronic GvHD, and – last but not least – characteristic histological findings in a liver biopsy [285]. It is important to note that, both clinically and histologically, transition between acute and chronic hepatic GvHD is gradual [255, 277].

6.2.1 Early Chronic GvHD of the Liver

Microscopically, the early phase of chronic hepatic GvHD is characterized by lymphoplasmacytic infiltration of the portal triads and more or less extensive destruction of small interlobular bile ducts (Fig. 6.3; [63, 176]). Often the number of bile ducts is decreased [37]. A prominent feature of chronic hepatic GvHD is cholestasis, which occurs in 80% of patients [63]. The portal infiltrates, in addition to lymphocytes and plasma cells, may contain a few eosinophils and neutrophils [277]. Remarkably, the inflammatory cellular infiltration in chronic hepatic GvHD can be more intense than in acute GvHD [76]. This most likely correlates with the hematological and immunological reconstitution of patients.

6.2.2 Late Chronic GvHD of the Liver

In the later stages of the disease, frequently, a definite loss of bile ducts and a marked fibrosis is observed (Fig. 6.4; [37, 286]). In fact the histomorphological picture of chronic hepatic GvHD may resemble primary biliary cirrhosis (PBC [37, 287]). In contrast to PBC and other chronic inflammatory processes chronic hepatic GvHD only rarely progresses to liver cirrhosis [253]. Nevertheless, to prevent irreversible damage and to start therapy in time, it is important to diagnose hepatic GvHD as early as possible [76].

6.2.3 Severity of Chronic GvHD of the Liver

There are considerable differences in the severity and extent of pathological changes in chronic hepatic GvHD. The severity of bile duct damage, of inflammation, and of portal fibrosis not only varies from patient to patient but also may vary in one and the same liver biopsy from one portal tract to another. Such variation in the severity and number of lesions can cause considerable sampling error and make interpretation of liver biopsies difficult [63].

6.2.4 Time Course of Chronic GvHD of the Liver

Little information appears in the literature on the time course of chronic hepatic GvHD. With increasing time there seems to be a progressive portal fibrosis and ductopenia [63, 176], but, as mentioned previously, liver cirrhosis results only rarely [176]. The indicators of activity and progression in chronic hepatic GvHD correspond to those in acute GvHD.

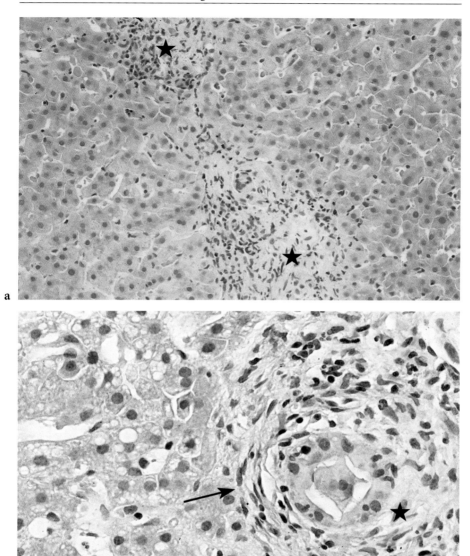

Fig. 6.3 a, b. Chronic GvHD of the liver, early phase. Lymphoplasmacytic infiltration of portal triads with destruction of small bile ducts and marked fibrosis (*asterisks*). Histological picture resembling PBC (*arrow*). **a** Biopsy of a 15-year-old male patient with AA obtained $3^{1}/_{2}$ months after HLA-identical allogeneic BMT. Chronic GvHD of the skin was also present. **b** Biopsy of a 1-year-old male infant with SCID obtained $6^{1}/_{2}$ months after HLA-nonidentical allogeneic BMT. Chronic GvHD of the skin was also present. H & E, **a** ×210, **b** ×420

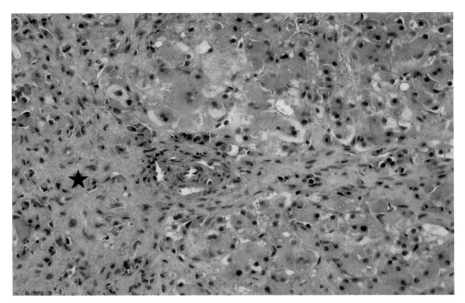

Fig. 6.4. Chronic GvHD of the liver, late phase. Marked fibrosis of parenchyma (*asterisk*) with loss of small bile ducts (ductopenic type of GvHD). No appreciable inflammatory infiltration. Biopsy of the same patient as in Fig. 5.14 obtained 6 months after BMT. van Gieson, ×210

6.2.5 Differential Diagnosis of Chronic GvHD of the Liver

The closest histomorphological similarity is between chronic hepatic GvHD and PBC [37, 287]. Apart from the unlikelihood of a coincidence of PBC and GvHD, such differential diagnosis can be resolved histologically. In contrast to PBC, chronic hepatic GvHD spares large bile ducts, shows no granulomata, and rarely if ever progresses to liver cirrhosis [253, 278]. Another potential differential diagnosis is chronic viral hepatitis, in particular hepatitis C (Table 6.2). Although there may be a considerable overlap in the histomorphology of the two disease entities, the presence of bile ducts with epithelial dysplasia and destruction favors chronic GvHD [286].

A diagnostic problem that cannot be settled by histology arises if hepatic GvHD coexists with hepatitis C [278]. Such simultaneous occurrence of GvHD and viral infection is of considerable clinical significance in patients after allogeneic HSCT and has been observed not only in the liver but also in the gut [270, 277]. Under these circumstances a reliable diagnosis can be made only by the combined application of clinical, serological, virological, and histomorphological methods. Difficulties may arise also if chronic GvHD must be distinguished from drug-induced liver damage [255].

Table 6.2. Differential diagnosis of chronic GvHD of the liver

1. Chronic viral hepatitis, e. g., by HCV
2. Chronic drug-induced liver damage
3. Primary biliary cirrhosis (PBC)

HCV, hepatitis C virus.

Although there is some overlap in the histomorphological picture of these disease processes, the key features of hepatic GvHD, the small bile duct lesions just described, can serve as a reliable discriminator [63].

6.2.6 Histodiagnostic Criteria of Chronic GvHD of the Liver

Epithelial atypia, destruction and loss of small interlobular bile ducts in association with portal inflammatory infiltrates primarily composed of lymphocytes and plasma cells are characteristic but not pathognomonic of chronic hepatic GvHD. Nor are cholestasis and other nonspecific histopathological findings. Inflammatory infiltrates in the liver tissue are frequently more pronounced than in acute hepatic GvHD. When needle biopsy specimens are evaluated histologically it is important to take into consideration the patchy distribution of bile duct lesions. By serial sections one often can avoid false-negative results.

6.3 Histological Features of Chronic GvHD of the Gastrointestinal Tract

In contrast to acute GvHD, chronic GvHD of the GIT has little influence on survival [176, 255]. Approximately 30% of patients with chronic GvHD show some kind of gastrointestinal involvement [253]. However, neither the stomach nor the gut are severely injured. In the past the esophagus was the organ most frequently damaged by chronic GvHD, with esophagitis, strictures, and obstruction [176, 211, 298]. Since the introduction of modern immunosuppression for GvHD prophylaxis, involvement of the esophagus has become rare [255].

6.3.1 Histopathology of Chronic GvHD of the Gastrointestinal Tract

Chronic GvHD of the GIT shows rather nonspecific pathological changes. In the small and large bowel, there is fibrosis of the submucosa sometimes accompanied by variable numbers of lymphocytes and plasma cells in the lamina propria [291, 325]. In contrast to acute GvHD, no ulceration of the intestinal mucosa is usually found [285, 298]. Frequently the mucosa shows structural distortion, focal atrophy, single apoptotic crypt epithelia, and signs of increased regeneration (Fig. 6.5). Rarely, the pathological changes result in formation of stricturing and obstruction [293].

6.3.2 Severity of Chronic GvHD of the Gastrointestinal Tract

Manifestations of chronic GvHD in the gut including functional disturbances are infrequent and mild. As mentioned before. the only previous exception to this rule was the esophagus.

6.3.3 Time Course of Chronic GvHD of the Gastrointestinal Tract

As determined by endoscopic biopsies, the colonic mucosa of patients 6 months after allogeneic BMT and subsequent acute GvHD shows only slight histopathological changes [17]. There is mild architectural distortion of the mucosa with crypt branching and villiform surface projections (Fig. 6.6). The lamina propria may be hypo- or hypercellular. Florid inflammation as in acute GvHD is rarely observed [17].

6.3.4 Differential Diagnosis of Chronic GvHD of the Gastrointestinal Tract

The three major causes of injury to the GIT after allogeneic HSCT are chemoradiation, infection, and GvHD [17]. Damage to the gut by chemotherapy or radiation primarily occurs in the first 3–4 weeks after transplantation. Intestinal infections may develop any time after transplant and primarily must be identified or ruled out by microbiology. If there is evidence of GvHD-induced dysmotility or stricturing, a full-thickness biopsy of the gut may yield appropriate diagnostic information [293]. A like examination may distinguish between scleroderma and GvHD of the esophagus. While fibrosis of the submucosa is characteristic of chronic GvHD, scleroderma shows submucosal as well as muscular fibrosis [176]. It should be evident from Table 6.3 that scleroderma does not represent a true differential diagnosis of chronic GvHD of the GIT.

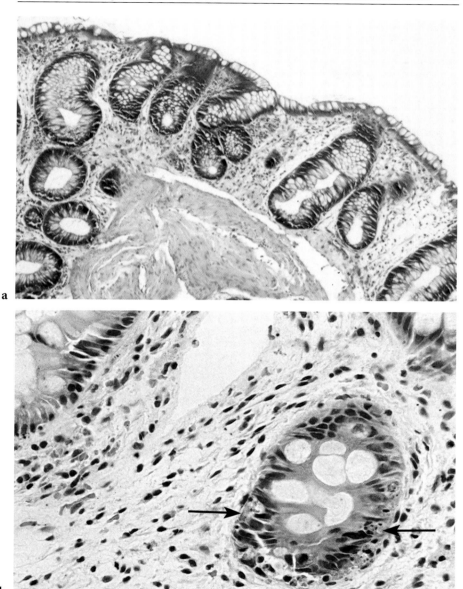

Fig. 6.5 a, b. Low-grade chronic GvHD of the colon. Slight structural distortion of crypts. Sparse lymphocytic infiltration of the lamina propria. Focally increased number of apoptotic crypt cells (*arrows*). Biopsy of an 8-year-old female patient with FA obtained 4 months after HLA-identical unrelated allogeneic BMT. Acute GvHD of the skin was present previously. H & E, **a** × 105, **b** × 420

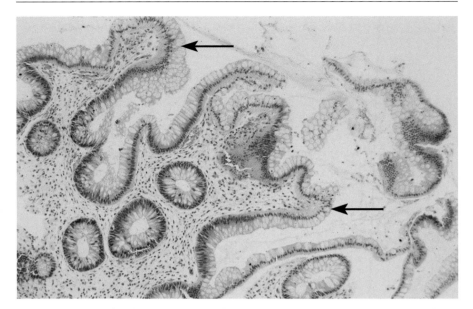

Fig. 6.6. Low-grade chronic GvHD of the colon. Architectural distortion of the mucosa with villiform surface projections (*arrows*). No signs of disease activity. Biopsy of the same patient as in Fig. 6.5. H&E, × 105

Table 6.3. Differential diagnosis of chronic GvHD of the gastrointestinal tract

1. Chronic viral enteritis, e.g., by CMV
2. Sequelae of chemoradiation damage of GIT
3. Chronic bacterial or fungal enteritis

CMV, cytomegalovirus; GIT, gastrointestinal tract.

6.3.5 Histodiagnostic Criteria of Chronic GvHD of the Gastrointestinal Tract

The basic pathology of chronic GvHD of the GIT is fibrosis of the submucosa. Since this cannot be assessed by mucosal biopsies, such biopsies are of limited value for the diagnosis of chronic GvHD [293]. Only if focal florid inflammation of the mucosa superimposes on the submucosal fibrosis might a mucosal biopsy be worthwhile. Otherwise a full-thickness biopsy of the gut is required.

6.4 Histological Features of Chronic GvHD of Other Organs

In addition to the three major target organs – skin, liver, and GIT – numerous other organs and tissues can be affected by chronic GvHD. As stated before, often it is difficult to prove that the lesions observed are in fact induced by GvHD and not some other pathogenetic mechanism. This might explain partially why many lesions ascribed to chronic GvHD, outside its classic target organs, appear histomorphologically heterogeneous and scarcely characteristic. That is to say, some of these pathological conditions may have been misinterpreted as chronic GvHD.

6.4.1 Histopathology of Chronic GvHD of the Oral Cavity and Eyes

Many patients with extensive chronic GvHD show an involvement of the mouth (40 % – 70 %) and eyes (up to 80 %; [176, 253]). In the buccal or labial mucosa lichen planus-like eruptions can be observed [115, 174] that histo-

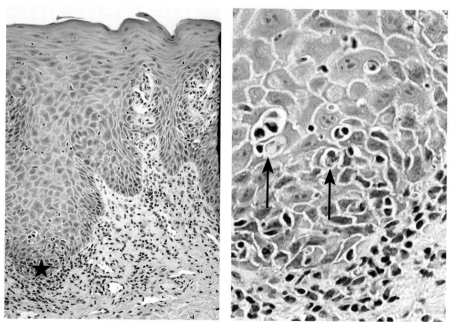

a   b

Fig. 6.7 a, b. Chronic GvHD of the buccal mucosa. Lymphoplasmacytic infiltration of the upper lamina propria with focal invasion of the basal epithelial layers (*asterisk*). Single apoptotic bodies (*arrows*). Biopsy of a 42-year-old male patient with CML obtained 7 months after allogeneic BMT. H & E, **a** × 120, **b** × 420

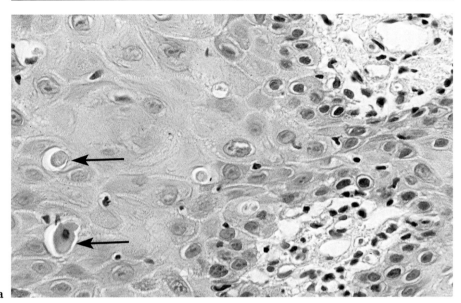

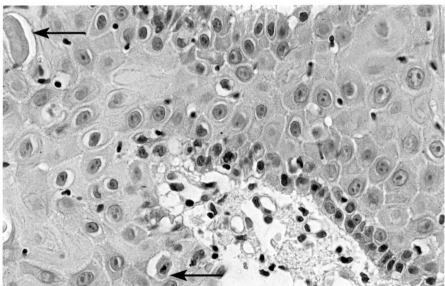

Fig. 6.8 a, b. Chronic GvHD of the oral mucosa. Tangential section of a biopsy from the inner lower lip. Sparse lymphocytic infiltration of the lamina propria and the squamous epithelium. Several apoptotic bodies (*arrows*). Biopsy of a 22-year-old male patient with AUL obtained $3^1/_2$ months after allogeneic BMT. Chronic GvHD of the skin and liver were also present. H & E, × 420

logically disclose a band-like mononuclear infiltrate in the superficial lamina propria with focal invasion of the basal epithelial layer and apoptosis of single cells [255]. A corresponding lesion is depicted in Fig. 6.7.

About 80% of patients with extensive chronic GvHD exhibit a sicca syndrome that may involve mouth, eyes, nose, and airways [277]. The salivary and lacrimal glands histologically show a diffuse infiltration by lymphocytes and plasma cells with fibrosis, atrophy, and destruction [148]. Ocular manifestations of chronic GvHD can include lymphoplasmacellular keratoconjunctivitis.

Since the diagnosis of chronic GvHD is based on clinical as well as histological criteria and since oral involvement is frequent, biopsies from the inner lower lip of patients play an important role in establishing the diagnosis and assessing the activity of the disease (Fig. 6.8; [176]). In this context it is stressed that 94%–100% of patients with a positive oral or labial biopsy show involvement of other organs [277]. If chronic GvHD is suspected, an oral or labial biopsy is accordingly recommended.

6.4.2 Histopathology of Chronic GvHD of the Lung

While the controversies concerning the existence of *acute* pulmonary GvHD persist, today the existence of *chronic* GvHD of the lung is largely accepted [84, 240, 277, 278]. The lesion most widely agreed to represent a morphological correlate of or, more precisely, a sequel to chronic GvHD is bronchiolitis obliterans (Fig. 6.9). This lesion, observed in about 10% of patients with chronic GvHD [70], frequently occurs simultaneously with chronic GvHD of extrathoracic sites [71, 255, 277, 278]. Bronchiolitis obliterans is thus a late event in chronic GvHD and by no means pathognomonic [176]. Lymphocytic bronchitis, by clinicians often ascribed to chronic GvHD, falls into the same category and by most pathologists is considered nonspecific [277]. In this context it is important to note that those who accept the existence of pulmonary GvHD do not claim that the lesions observed are histomorphologically specific [351].

6.4.3 Histopathology of Chronic GvHD of the Bone Marrow and Lymphatic Organs

There are several possibilities how chronic GvHD can impair hematopoiesis [133]. Bone marrow, lymph nodes, spleen, and thymus are major targets for GvHD [255]. As a result of damage by chronic GvHD, these organs histologically show varying degrees of lymphocyte depletion (Fig. 6.10) and atrophy (Fig. 6.11). Severe immunodeficiency or aplastic anemia can be the aftermath [19]. However, in the individual patient other pathomechanisms

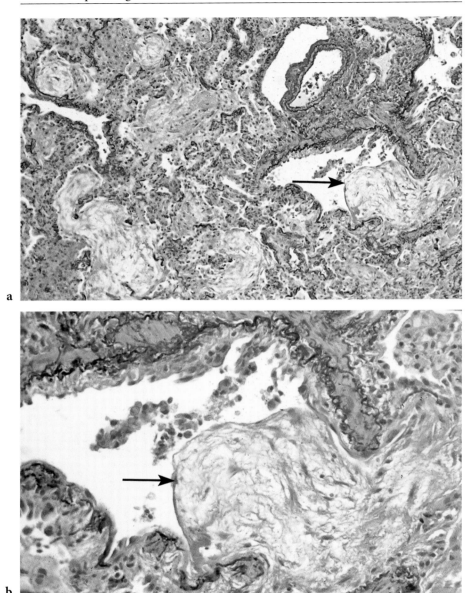

a

b

Fig. 6.9a, b. Bronchiolitis obliterans in chronic GvHD. Fibrosing granulation tissue plugging the lumen of bronchioli (*arrows*). No lymphocytic infiltration of the pulmonary tissue. Biopsy of a 19-year-old male patient with AUL obtained 8 months after HLA-identical allogeneic BMT. Chronic GvHD of the skin and liver were also present. Elastica-van Gieson, **a** ×105, **b** ×210

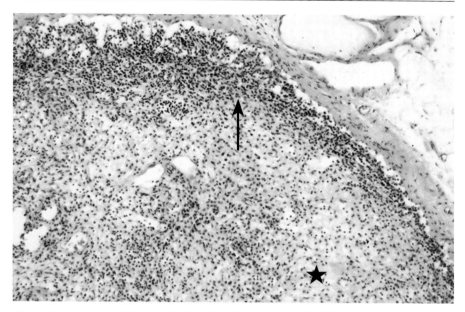

Fig. 6.10. Lymph node atrophy in chronic GvHD. Marked lymphocytic depletion (*asterisk*). Some residual lymphocytes in the subcapsular cortical region (*arrow*). Post mortem finding in a 52-year-old male patient with CML 10 months after allogeneic BMT. Extensive chronic GvHD of the skin was also present. H&E, ×105

besides GvHD may be active in causing immunologic or hematopoietic insufficiency [142, 278, 306]. Consequently, the histopathological changes shown in Figs. 6.10 and 6.11 basically could be caused by different pathogenic mechanisms.

Finally, patients with chronic GvHD frequently show signs of autoimmunity [70], probably induced by damage to the thymus during acute GvHD [283]. To give an example, among many other autoimmune diseases polymyositis has been observed as a sequel to chronic GvHD [241]. The histomorphology of this disease shows no features characteristic of GvHD, but a picture identical to idiopathic polymyositis [241].

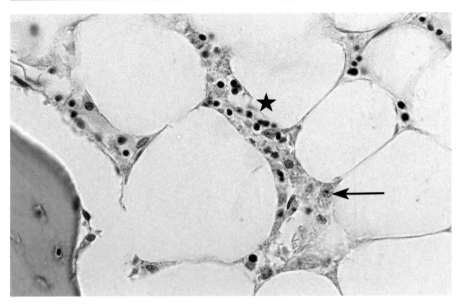

Fig. 6.11. Bone marrow aplasia in chronic GvHD. Complete loss of hematopoiesis. There are only single lymphoid cells (*asterisk*) and siderophages (*arrow*) in the medullary stroma. Post mortem finding in the same patient as in Fig. 6.10. H & E, × 420

6.5 Histological Grading of Chronic GvHD

There is no generally accepted histological grading system for chronic GvHD. The histomorphological assessment of lesions in chronic GvHD is primarily used for diagnostic purposes, and mainly clinical criteria are employed for grading. The clinicopathological classification system shown in Table 4.3 is based on a combination of clinical and histological findings [255, 305]. There is a close correlation between the three grades of severity defined by the classification used in Table 4.3 and the prognosis of patients with chronic GvHD [176].

Risk factors for chronic GvHD, as already mentioned, are preceding acute GvHD and positive skin or lip biopsy at 3 months after allogeneic HSCT [176]. When a skin or oral biopsy is positive in a patient with subclinical chronic GvHD and GvHD prophylaxis has been discontinued, about 70 % of patients will develop overt chronic disease within the next few months. While patients with limited chronic GvHD usually have a good prognosis, the course is frequently unfavorable for those with extensive disease [176]. Consequently, the clinicopathological assessment of chronic GvHD possesses a considerable prognostic significance.

7 Immunohistological Features of GvHD

From the foregoing discussion of the histomorphology of GvHD it is evident that a certain number of differential diagnostic problems cannot be resolved by routine histology. One asks whether some of these questions can be answered by immunohistology, proven to be a valuable diagnostic aid in other fields of pathology such as the typing of tumors or of glomerulonephritis [60].

Do immunohistological markers permit:

1. The confirmation of GvHD histodiagnosis?
2. The early diagnosis of acute GvHD?
3. The clarification of GvHD differential diagnosis?

Since the present monograph is focused on the clinical and diagnostic pathology of GvHD, the findings presented are exclusively based on the study of formalin-fixed paraffin-embedded tissues as employed in routine pathology. This applies to the published data referred to as well as the immunohistological investigations performed. One should thus be assured that the findings reported are relevant to the clinical and diagnostic pathology in man.

Assessment of immunohistological markers in formalin-fixed paraffin-embedded tissues has become possible since monoclonal antibodies, able to detect antigenic epitopes in such tissue specimens, are available [34]. In spite of the many morphological studies performed, no immunohistological marker has yet been introduced into the routine diagnosis of GvHD. It is time to summarize the data collected, define the immunohistological correlates of acute and chronic GvHD and, last but not least, determine if immunohistological parameters can assist in the diagnosis of GvHD.

Before addressing these issues, one should remember that the diagnostic value of immunohistochemistry is a topic of general importance in pathology. A recent statement by a respected pathologist perfectly characterizes the situation: "… it has been my experience when dealing with a considerable amount of referred material that if I was not able to make a diagnosis on H&E sections it was only very rarely that diagnostic clarification was achieved by immunocytochemistry" [111]. With respect to topics such as inflammation many pathologists would agree, but definitely not with regard to tumor pathology. The question remains whether or not the above statement holds true for GvHD?

Starting points for an immunohistological analysis of GvHD lesions can be:

1. Immunophenotypic characterization of the inflammatory infiltrate by markers such as CD3, CD20, CD4, CD8, CD57, CD68, CD1a [15, 165, 167]
2. Immunohistological determination of selective markers of effector cells such as TIA-1, HECA-452 or GMP-17 [21, 67, 276]
3. Immunohistochemical assessment of surface molecules of epithelial target cells such as HLA-DR or ICAM-1 [291]

Within the past two decades these and other aspects of GvHD have been studied immunohistologically. However, the purpose of most investigations has not been to evaluate the diagnostic potential but to determine the possible pathogenic role of the respective factors in the development of GvHD.

7.1 Immunohistological Features of Acute GvHD of the Skin

Most data published on the immunohistochemistry of acute GvHD are concerned with findings in the skin. There are several reasons for this: the skin is the organ most often involved by GvHD; in the course of the disease the skin is affected first; skin biopsies are easy to obtain and do not endanger patients; skin biopsies can be repeated without difficulty; the immunohistological features of the skin are the best for correlation with gross and microscopic findings. Finally, when a skin rash appears in a patient after allogeneic HSCT it is normally desirable to clarify the diagnosis as rapidly as possible.

7.1.1 Immunophenotype of the Inflammatory Infiltrate

The many immunohistological studies performed within the past 20 years unanimously indicate that the inflammatory infiltrate of acute GvHD lesions primarily consists of lymphocytes carrying the pan-T-cell marker CD3 (Fig. 7.1; [165, 172, 198, 217]). These T-lymphocytes belong to the CD8$^+$ as well as the CD4$^+$ subset [12, 173].

Today, these T-cell subtypes can no longer be interpreted as having discrete functions – e.g., CD4$^+$ = T-helper cells, CD8$^+$ = T cytotoxic/suppressor cells – since basically both are able to exert both functions [191]. In acute GvHD of skin both T-cell subsets can occur in the dermis as well as in the epidermis [15, 80, 198]. However, there is evidence that in fully established GvHD lesions CD8$^+$ T-cells predominate in the epidermis (Fig. 7.2) whereas CD4$^+$ T-cells predominate in the dermis [55, 95].

These observations are supported by the briefly described immunohistological study that follows (for details see pp. 127–128). Skin biopsies of 60 patients with GvHD grade II–III and of 41 patients with non-GvHD inflammatory skin lesions (controls) were screened for CD3$^+$, CD8$^+$, and OPD4$^+$ T-lym-

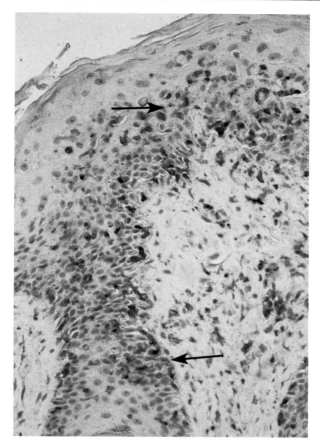

Fig. 7.1. Acute GvHD of the skin. Diffuse infiltration of the lower epidermis and the upper parts of the hair follicle by CD3$^+$ T-lymphocytes (*arrows*). Biopsy of a 16-year-old male patient with AML obtained 53 days after HLA-identical unrelated allogeneic BMT. CD3-immunohistology, ×210

phocytes, CD57$^+$ NK-cells, CD68$^+$ macrophages, CD1a$^+$ Langerhans' cells, and CD20$^+$ B-cells. The marker OPD4, which primarily but not exclusively reacts with CD4$^+$ T-cells [89], had to be used since CD4 specific monoclonal antibodies applicable for the detection of CD4 antigen in formalin-fixed paraffin-embedded tissue are not yet available. The results obtained are still valid since the predominant localization of OPD4$^+$ T-lymphocytes in the dermis in acute GvHD [55, 67] has also been observed in the present studies (Fig. 7.3).

A summary of some of the immunohistological findings is shown in Fig. 7.4. As is evident CD3$^+$ T-cells are present in the epidermis of practically

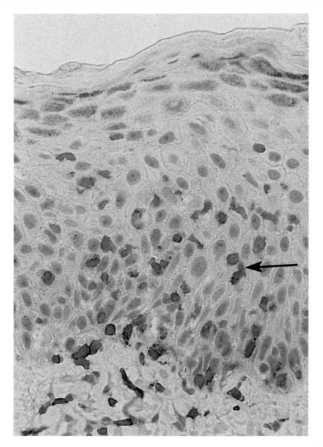

Fig. 7.2. Acute GvHD of the skin. Infiltration of the epidermis by CD8⁺ T-lympho-cytes (*arrow*). Biopsy of a 16-year-old male patient with MDS obtained 57 days after HLA-identical unrelated allogeneic PBSCT. CD8-immunohistology, ×420

all GvHD lesions (97%). In contrast, there is no significant difference in the occurrence of CD3⁺ T-cells in the dermis of GvHD lesions and controls. Similarly, CD8⁺ T-cells are present in the epidermis of about 95% of the GvHD skin lesions whereas there is no unequivocal difference in CD8⁺ T-cells in the dermis of GvHD and control lesions. Finally, while OPD4⁺ T-cells occur in the epidermis of only 35% of GvHD lesions, they are present within the dermis in more than 90%. Once more, there is no significant difference in the dermal infiltration by OPD4⁺ T-cells between GvHD and control lesions (Fig. 7.4).

This study confirms the marked epidermotropism of T-lymphocytes in acute GvHD. In addition it corroborates published data on the different

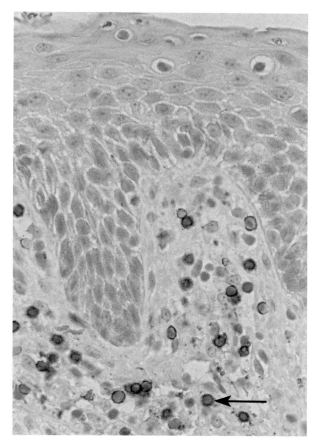

Fig. 7.3. Acute GvHD of the skin. Infiltration of the upper dermis by OPD4⁺ T-lymphocytes (*arrow*). Biopsy of a 3 ¹/₂-month-old male infant with SCID and intrauterine MFT. OPD4-immunohistology, × 420

localization of CD8⁺ and OPD4⁺ T-cells in GvHD skin lesions[55, 95, 168, 239]. It should also be noted that skin-homing memory T-cells [38] recognized by the OPD4 antibody most likely participate in the development of the skin lesions of acute GvHD. From the data shown in Fig. 7.4 it is obvious that only the study of lymphocytic infiltrates in the epidermis is diagnostically useful. In contrast, the immunophenotypic analysis of dermal infiltrates appears irrelevant.

The selective localization of CD8⁺ and CD4⁺ or OPD4⁺ T-cells within different compartments of the skin cannot be considered a permanent feature of acute cutaneous GvHD. It may well be a transient phenomenon only in fully developed lesions [95]. Unfortunately, there are no studies on the

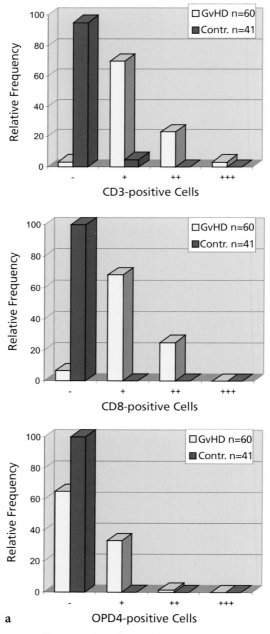

Fig. 7.4a, b. Summary of immunohistological findings in skin biopsies of 60 patients with acute GvHD and 41 patients with non-GvHD inflammatory skin lesions (controls). Results of the epidermis (**a**) and the dermis (**b**) are shown separately. For interpretation of findings see text. The support of Dr. E. Bachstein, Ulm/Kempten, in preparing this figure is grateful acknowledged

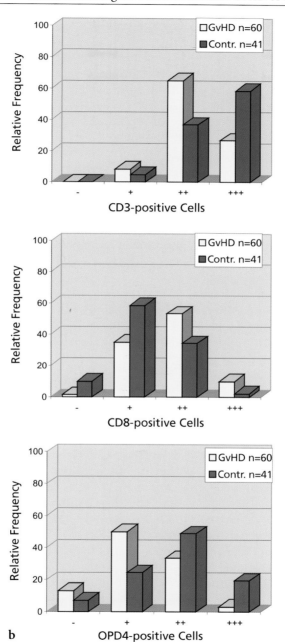

Fig. 7.4 b. Legend see p. 108

development of acute GvHD using immunohistology for analysis of sequential skin biopsies.

Inflammatory diseases were originally subdivided, according to the prevalence of T-cell subsets, into two groups: (1) diseases with CD4[+] T-cell dominance and (2) diseases with CD8[+] T-cell dominance. GvHD was assumed to belong to the latter group [167]. It has become obvious that the situation is more complex. Yet it still holds true that classic delayed hypersensitivity reactions are primarily mediated by CD4[+] T-lymphocytes [64] whereas cytolytic T-cell reactions are mostly mediated by CD8[+] T-lymphocytes [191].

By routine histology or immunohistochemistry it is impossible to distinguish host-derived and donor-derived cells within GvHD lesions. Using in situ hybridization (IHS) with a Y-chromosome-specific probe, it has been shown in the sex-mismatched constellation that a significant portion (45%–90%) of both CD8[+] and CD4[+] T-lymphocytes found in acute GvHD skin lesions are donor-derived [20, 316]. The Y-chromosome-positive donor cells appear in lesional skin approximately two weeks after allogeneic HSCT, correlating in number with GvHD severity [156]. While there are only few donor cells in early acute GvHD, the majority of T-lymphocytes in fully established lesions are donor-derived. The T-cells within lesional skin, as outlined previously, possess anti-host cytotoxic activity [171].

NK-cells also are frequently present in acute GvHD of skin [2, 15, 80, 254]. Since NK-cells lack an epitope-directed receptor, they cannot be involved in the induction of acute GvHD [177]. NK-cells recruited nonspecifically may nonetheless contribute to the manifestation of GvHD lesions [156, 177, 254]. Most of the NK-cells express CD57 antigen (Fig. 7.5). However, only about 50% of the GvHD skin lesions studied showed a CD57[+] NK-cell infiltration of the epidermis. The other 50% reacted negative.

Cells derived from the monocyte–macrophage lineage are regularly present in GvHD skin lesions. Very likely most of them serve as scavenger macrophages for the local uptake and degradation of cellular debris. By immunohistology it can be shown that these cells, occurring in the epidermis as well as the dermis, express CD68 antigen (Fig. 7.6). In the present study CD68[+] macrophages were detected in all GvHD skin lesions (100%).

Another cellular component of the inflammatory infiltrates in acute cutaneous GvHD are Langerhans' cells. They can be identified immunohistologically using CD1a as a marker. Most published work indicates that the number of epidermal Langerhans' cells in acute GvHD, as compared to normal controls, is reduced significantly [83, 88, 95, 349]. This most likely is not due to GvHD but to toxic effects of the pretransplant conditioning regimen [95, 311]. The only exception to this rule might be in inborn immunodeficiencies such as RD which lack Langerhans' cells a priori [91]. For the rest, the present immunohistological studies completely confirm the reported reduction of CD1a[+] Langerhans' cells in acute cutaneous GvHD.

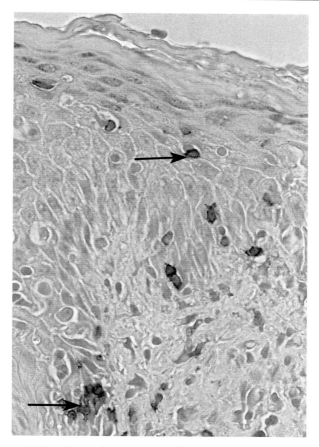

Fig. 7.5. Acute GvHD of the skin. Sparse infiltration of the papillary dermis and the epidermis by CD57⁺-NK cells (*arrows*). Biopsy of the same patient as in Fig. 7.2. CD57-immunohistology, × 420

B-cells usually don't belong to the inflammatory infiltrate of acute GvHD skin lesions [15, 80, 95, 172]. This is not specific for acute GvHD but also a finding in other types of acute dermatitis [3]. In any event, in the study described here all the GvHD skin biopsies examined for CD20⁺ B-cells gave a negative result. This is in keeping with the idea that acute GvHD represents a cell mediated immunopathological reaction.

Like many other inflammatory skin diseases, acute cutaneous GvHD shows a cellular infiltrate with a prominent CD4⁺/CD8⁺ T-cell component [236, 256]. There is a considerable overlap in the immunohistological features of acute GvHD and drug eruptions, erythema multiforme, and atopic dermatitis [83, 92]. It is noteworthy that in acute GvHD the lympho-

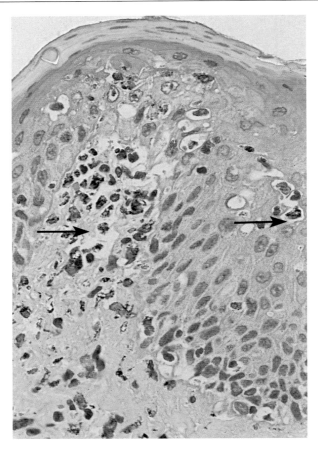

Fig. 7.6. Acute GvHD of the skin. Focal infiltration of the epidermis and the upper dermis by CD68⁺ macrophages (*arrows*). Biopsy of the same patient as in Fig. 5.17, but taken 55 days after BMT. CD68-immunohistology, × 420

cytes show a tendency to infiltrate the epidermis and that, in fully established GvHD, CD8⁺ T-cells, at least at times, predominate intraepidermally.

The local activity of alloreactive T-cells and/or cytokines leads to the recruitment of accessory cells, finally resulting in a complex inflammatory infiltrate [97]. This scenario becomes even more evident if one remembers that the GvHD infiltrate is composed not only of specifically targeted and nonspecifically recruited accessory cells, but also consists of both donor and host cells. This latter feature best characterizes the complexity and peculiarity of GvHD lesions: local presence and interaction of cells from two different individuals.

7.1.2 Selective Markers of Effector Cells

A number of investigators have tried to employ more specific markers for the immunohistological recognition of GvHD lesions. The mouse monoclonal antibody TIA-1 identifies cytotoxic T-lymphocytes (CTLs) by reaction with a RNA-binding nucleolysin protein [276]. Using this marker CTLs can be detected immunohistologically in acute GvHD lesions of skin and lip [274, 276]. Since TIA-1$^+$ CTLs can also, however, be observed in drug reactions and GvHD-like autoimmune skin lesions [168],TIA-1 is not a specific marker for acute GvHD.

This lack of specificity is also evident from immunohistological studies on intraepidermal lymphocytes in psoriatic lesions. CD8$^+$ T-cells, CTLs, and NK-cells are characterized by cytoplasmic granules containing the cytotoxic proteins GMP-17 (p15-TIA-1), perforin, and granzyme B [21]. GMP-17$^+$ cells are present in the epidermis of acute GvHD skin lesions. In psoriasis a substantial infiltration of lesional skin by CD8$^+$ and CD4$^+$ T-cells is observed. These lymphocytes also express GMP-17 [21]. Therefore, the immunohistological assessment of GMP-17 does not discriminate between psoriasis and acute GvHD.

HECA-452 is a rat monoclonal antibody recognizing lymphocytes with skin-homing properties [67]. Such cells are capable of a rapid site-specific accumulation. Acute GvHD of skin and erythema multiforme share many clinical and histological features. Immunophenotypically the two diseases are essentially indistinguishable as well. Both types of skin lesions contain OPD4$^+$ T-lymphocytes predominantly confined to the dermis, whereas HECA-452$^+$ T-cells, mostly CD8$^+$, concentrate in the epidermis [67]. Consequently, the HECA-452 antibody does not immunohistologically discriminate between erythema multiforme and acute GvHD. Nor does the skin-homing T-cell subset, defined by the adhesion receptor CLA (cutaneous lymphocyte-associated antigen), which besides occurring in acute GvHD is found in atopic dermatitis and other inflammatory skin diseases [38, 85, 256].

7.1.3 Markers of Epithelial Target Cells

Expression of HLA-DR by keratinocytes appears to be an early feature of acute GvHD [235, 309, 311]. While most investigators regard HLA-DR expression by epidermal cells, prior to lymphocytic infiltration, a necessary step in the development of acute GvHD [12, 14, 291, 292, 325], some do not [32]. These latter authors observed HLA-DR$^+$ as well as HLA-DR$^-$ acute GvHD. HLA-DR$^-$ lesions were most often found in patients receiving CSA prophylaxis, strongly suggesting modification of GvHD immunohistology by medication. In follow-up biopsies HLA-DR$^-$ acute GvHD frequently turned into HLA-DR$^+$ acute GvHD [32]. Notwithstanding the correctness of these observations, it is a fact that HLA-DR is expressed by keratinocytes and other epithelial cells in toxic as well as infectious lesions [12]. Accordingly, HLA-DR fails to qualify as a marker for acute GvHD.

Formation of intercellular adhesion molecules (ICAM) such as ICAM-1 by keratinocytes is significantly increased during acute GvHD [291, 325]. Likewise is the expression of vascular cell adhesion molecules (VCAM) such as VCAM-1 on dendritic cells and macrophages [235]. It is known that these molecules, like substances heretofore described, are produced not only in acute GvHD but also in the course of completely different pathological processes [12, 334]. The diagnostic value of the immunohistological assessment here is unclear.

7.1.4 Immunohistological Differential Diagnosis of Acute GvHD of the Skin

Histomorphologically, acute GvHD of the skin is a lymphocytic interface dermatitis with scattered apoptotic bodies in the epidermis. Immunohistologically, it represents a T-cell mediated inflammatory skin disease that shares many features with cell-mediated immunopathological reactions [191] as well as diseases such as atopic dermatitis [85, 256], erythema multiforme and discoid lupus erythematosus [3], mycosis fungoides [236], viral infections of skin [167], and drug-induced dermatitis [83, 238].

When the actual situation of patients who are at risk of developing acute GvHD is taken into consideration, then cutaneous drug eruptions of the interface type and viral infections of skin, e.g., by HSV or VZV, are of particular importance in the differential diagnosis [3, 227]. Depending on the stage of development, these skin lesions may show a close immunohistological similarity to acute GvHD. Inflammatory infiltrates composed of $CD3^+$, $CD4^+$, $CD8^+$ T-lymphocytes, and NK-cells, increased expression of HLA-DR, ICAM-1, VCAM-1, and other activation or adhesion molecules can occur in all these skin lesions. No single immunohistological marker or marker pattern on its own is specific for acute GvHD [227, 325]. However, if the clinical context and the histomorphological findings are taken into account, then certain immunophenotypical markers can be useful diagnostically.

Table 7.1 summarizes the immunohistological findings in acute GvHD of the skin. In most instances the observations are in agreement with published data. Whether the lesions in other GvHD target organs show the same immunohistological characteristics remains to be seen.

The conclusions that can be drawn concerning the diagnostic value of immunohistological markers in acute GvHD of skin are listed in Table 7.2. Independent of all other aspects, the most important conclusion is that only immunohistological features of the epidermis are characteristic while findings in the dermis are not discriminatory.

Table 7.1. Immunohistological findings in grade II-III acute GvHD of the skin

1. Infiltration of the epidermis and dermis by CD3$^+$ T-cells
2. Infiltration of the epidermis predominantly by CD8$^+$ T-cells
3. Infiltration of the dermis predominantly by OPD4$^+$ T-cells
4. Absence of CD20$^+$ B-cells from the epidermis and dermis
5. Inconsistent infiltration of the epidermis by CD57$^+$ NK-cells
6. Strong infiltration of the epidermis and dermis by CD68$^+$ macrophages
7. Reduction of CD1a$^+$ Langerhans' cells in the epidermis

Table 7.2. Conclusions concerning the diagnostic value of immunohistological markers in acute GvHD of the skin

1. The epidermis is the primary target of alloreactive T-lymphocytes in acute GvHD.
2. The immunophenotype of lymphocytes in the epidermis only is important in acute GvHD.
3. The immunophenotypical analysis of lymphocytic infiltrates in the dermis is not informative.
4. No single immunohistological marker or marker pattern is pathognomonic for acute GvHD.
5. The combination of clinical, histomorphological, and immunohistological data can be helpful diagnostically.

7.2 Immunohistological Features of Acute GvHD of the Liver

The number of studies on the immunohistology of acute GvHD of the liver as compared to reports on acute GvHD of the skin is very small. In addition, the immunohistological analysis of hepatic GvHD is more difficult because of the inconsistency and uneven distribution of lesions in this organ. Published information on this topic is very limited.

7.2.1 Immunophenotype of the Inflammatory Infiltrate

Acute GvHD of the liver is characterized by a sparse to moderate portal infiltration of T-lymphocytes, macrophages, and CD57$^+$ NK-cells [291]. The T-cells infiltrate and destroy the epithelia of small intrahepatic bile ducts [314]. Immunohistologically, they primarily belong to the CD4$^+$ or OPD4$^+$

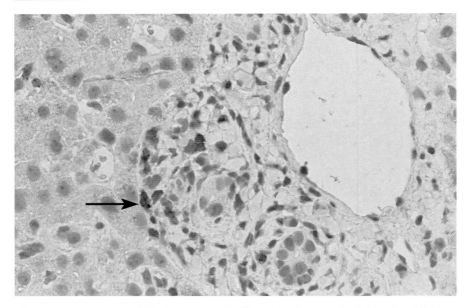

Fig. 7.7. Acute GvHD of the liver. Sparse infiltration of a portal triad by CD8$^+$ T-lymphocytes (*arrow*). Two small bile ducts are recognizable. Biopsy of a 13-year-old male patient with FA obtained 3 months after HLA-identical related allogeneic BMT. Acute GvHD of the skin was also present. CD8-immunohistology, $\times$420

subtype, to a lesser extent to the CD8$^+$ T-cell subset (Fig. 7.7; [63, 170, 213]). This pattern may change with time [314]. The portal infiltrates also contain macrophages and CD56$^+$ or CD57$^+$ NK-cells [170, 291]. B-cells are only rarely found in acute hepatic GvHD [63].

From the study of liver GvHD after sex-mismatched HSCT with Y-chromosome-specific ISH, it is known that the majority of T-lymphocytes present in hepatic lesions are donor-derived [9]. This is evidence that alloreactive donor T-cells in fact are active locally. It also indicates that Y-chromosome-specific ISH is a valuable tool for confirming the diagnosis of acute GvHD [9].

7.2.2 Selective Markers of Effector Cells

By immunolabeling with antibodies to GB4 (a serine protease present in the granules of activated T and NK-cells) most of the cytotoxic T-lymphocytes in hepatic GvHD lesions show signs of activation [170]. This again is not specific for GvHD.

7.2.3 Markers of Epithelial Target Cells

In the early stages of acute hepatic GvHD the bile duct epithelia, but not the hepatocytes [325], show an increased expression of HLA-DR [63, 213, 314]. Since this response can also be observed in primary biliary cirrhosis, it is not pathognomonic for GvHD [213].

7.2.4 Immunohistological Differential Diagnosis of Acute GvHD of the Liver

Several diseases immunohistologically resemble acute hepatic GvHD. These are autoimmune cholangitis (AIC), primary biliary cirrhosis (PBC), and occasionally viral hepatitis [87, 170]. Basically, an immunohistological similarity exists between acute GvHD of the liver and acute liver allograft rejection [249]. In practice a distinction of these two is not required since the liver itself is typically not involved when acute GvHD develops after allogeneic liver transplantation [59, 345]. There is evidence, however, that CD4$^+$ T-cells dominate in hepatic GvHD [170, 213] whereas CD8$^+$ T-cells play a major role in liver allograft rejection [249]. Since clearcut distinction of acute hepatic GvHD from AIC is not possible, and since distinction from PBC is feasible by other means (see p. 92), only viral hepatitis is important with regard to differential diagnosis.

The similar immunohistological pattern of hepatic GvHD and PBC possibly suggests a similar pathomechanism [213], namely, activity of alloreactive T-cells in GvHD and of autoreactive T-cells in PBC [63, 170].

7.2.5 Immunohistological Criteria of Acute GvHD of the Liver

The histomorphological picture of acute hepatic GvHD, as outlined before, is relatively characteristic. Regarding immunohistological criteria one might point out that:

1. The lymphocytic infiltration of portal triads and small bile ducts in particular includes CD4$^+$ or OPD4$^+$ T-cells.
2. CD20$^+$ B-cells are absent from liver tissue.

7.3 Immunohistological Features of Acute Gastrointestinal GvHD

Although the involvement of the GIT plays an important role in the clinicopathological manifestation of acute GvHD there are only few immunohistological studies on gastrointestinal GvHD. This may be due in part to the fact that the assessment of the GIT, with use of endoscopy and biopsy, is more complicated than that of the skin. Also, the histological as well as the immunohistological evaluation of gastrointestinal biopsies is more difficult because of the "physiological inflammation" of the intestinal mucosa. Approximately 70% of the T-lymphocytes normally present in the intestinal lamina propria carry the CD4 phenotype, while most of the intraepithelial T-lymphocytes carry the CD8 [342]. B-cells usually concentrate to the follicles. The normal presence of these cell types in the GIT, in contrast to their normal absence from skin and liver, complicates the evaluation.

7.3.1 Immunophenotype of the Inflammatory Infiltrate

If one takes into account the inherent difficulties associated with the immunohistological interpretation of gastrointestinal biopsies, it is not surprising that many findings reported are contradictory [198, 311]. However, most investigators agree that the number of intraepithelial CD8$^+$ T-lymphocytes is increased in acute GvHD of the GIT (Fig. 7.8; [87, 311, 325, 342]). It must be emphasized that donor-derived intraepithelial CD8$^+$ T-lymphocytes are present in destructive lesions of acute gastrointestinal GvHD [216]. Some authors also report an increased infiltration of the mucosa by CD4$^+$

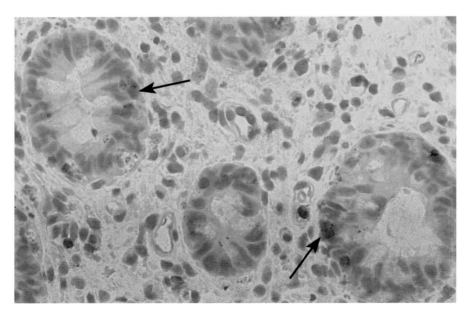

Fig. 7.8. Acute GvHD of the colon. Increased number of CD8$^+$ T-lymphocytes in crypt epithelium (*arrows*). Multiple apoptotic bodies are visible. Biopsy of the same patient as in Fig. 5.15. CD8-immunohistology, ×420

T-cells [87, 342]. No significant change has been observed with respect to NK-cells and macrophages [311, 325].

7.3.2 Selective Markers of Effector Cells

Activation markers of T-cells show no significant change in patients with acute GvHD of the rectal mucosa [311]. It is unknown if this finding is representative for gastrointestinal GvHD as a whole.

7.3.3 Markers of Epithelial Target Cells

In the early phase of acute GvHD of the GIT an increased expression of HLA-DR by enterocytes has been observed [216, 309, 311]. This is not a phenomenon characteristic for GvHD since it also occurs in other types of gastrointestinal damage.

7.3.4 Immunohistological Differential Diagnosis of Acute GvHD of the GIT

Immunohistological features resembling acute gastrointestinal GvHD have been observed in CMV infection of the GIT [86]. Clarification is possible by identifying CMV cells through immunohistochemistry (IHC) or ISH [22]. The histomorphological and immunohistological analysis may of course be more difficult when GvHD and CMV occur simultaneously [86].

7.4 Immunohistological Features of Acute GvHD of Other Organs

Several papers describe the immunohistological features of acute GvHD of the oral mucosa and salivary glands [349]. In most instances, the results of immunophenotypic analysis of inflammatory infiltrates in these lesions closely resemble findings in the skin, liver, and GIT. Biopsies from the oral mucosa or lower lip are diagnostically the most relevant [274].

7.5 Immunohistological Features of Chronic GvHD

In contrast to acute GvHD, relatively few studies have reported on the immunohistology of chronic GvHD. This may be due to the ease with which chronic GvHD can be diagnosed clinically and/or histologically in most instances. There is no need for these more complex diagnostic measures. It may be important to note that patients with chronic GvHD frequently

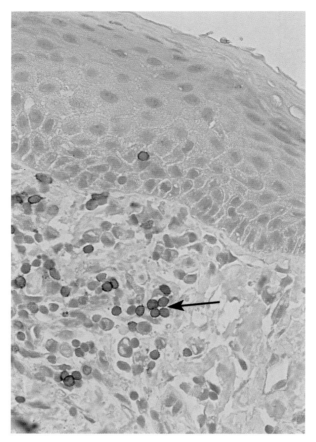

Fig. 7.9. Chronic GvHD of the skin, lichenoid type. Infiltration of the upper dermis by OPD4$^+$ T-lymphocytes (*arrow*). Biopsy of the same patient as in Fig. 6.1. OPD4-immunohistology, ×420

receive some kind of immunosuppressive treatment. This may considerably modify the immunohistological findings as well as the histopathology of lesions.

7.5.1 Immunohistological Features of Chronic GvHD of the Skin

Chronic cutaneous GvHD has been studied immunohistologically much less frequently than the acute variety [291]. This is particularly true for chronic sclerodermatous GvHD which lacks a distinct inflammatory infiltrate. Chronic GvHD of the lichenoid type is characterized by a bandlike infiltrate in the upper dermis; it contains CD3$^+$ T-cells but no B-cells [15]. In some immunohistological studies a predominance of CD8$^+$ over CD4$^+$ T-cells is reported in the dermal lymphocytic infiltrates [15, 115, 148]. Other studies indicate that CD4$^+$ or OPD4$^+$ (Fig. 7.9) can exceed CD8$^+$ T-lymphocytes [95, 198, 349]. Whatever the truth may be, more important than the question of which T-cell subset predominates is the observation that both T-cell types possess specific anti-host cytotoxicity [171].

Whereas chronic GvHD of the lichenoid type lacks CD20$^+$ B-cells, plasma cells are frequently present. Lesions also contain CD68$^+$ macrophages and melanophages. Interestingly, NK-cells usually are not detectable immunohistologically [15, 95].

In chronic cutaneous GvHD, focal infiltration of the basal layers of the epidermis by lymphocytes, sometimes accompanied by keratinocyte apoptosis, indicates activity and progression of the disease. These focal epidermotropic lymphocytic infiltrates usually consist of CD8$^+$ T-cells [95].

7.5.2 Immunohistological Features of Chronic GvHD of the Liver

In chronic GvHD of the liver an aberrant expression of MHC class II antigens by bile duct epithelial cells is evident [63]. Otherwise, immunohistological data on chronic hepatic GvHD are very sparse.

7.5.3 Immunohistological Features of Chronic Gastrointestinal GvHD

The large and small intestines are not consistantly and not severely injured by chronic GvHD. The gut exhibits nonspecific changes including submucosal fibrosis and increased infiltration by lymphocytes and plasma cells [291]. The few immunohistological data available are not particularly informative.

7.5.4 Immunohistological Features of Chronic GvHD of Other Organs

A predominance of CD8$^+$ over CD4$^+$ T-cells has been observed in lichenoid GvHD lesions of the oral mucosa [115, 148]. In contrast, in true lichen planus, histologically indistinguishable from the lichenoid type of chronic GvHD, CD4$^+$ exceed CD8$^+$ T-cells [149].

8 Conclusions

GvHD represents a unique immunopathological process induced by interaction of alloreactive T-lymphocytes with distinct target tissues. Nonimmunological factors are involved as well. GvHD affects many organs such as the skin, liver, and GIT and sometimes runs a devastating or even lethal course. GvHD may develop in different clinical settings such as blood transfusion, MFT, DLI, or SOT. However, most often it is observed as a complication of allogeneic BMT or PBSCT. In the latter case the histomorphology of lesions can be modified considerably by GvHD prophylaxis or treatment. This must be taken into account when analyzing the clinical and diagnostic pathology of GvHD today.

Understanding of the histomorphology of GvHD is considerably improved by knowledge of GvHD pathogenesis. Whereas the inductive phase is dominated by the immunologically specific action of alloreactive T-lymphocytes, in the effector phase nonspecific factors such as cytokines are also involved. In the analysis of GvHD lesions the identification of the immunospecific components (alloreactive T-cells) appears more important than the detection of the later nonspecific effects.

Before discussing the histopathology it should be pointed out that patients with GvHD may exhibit three different types of lesions: (1) histomorphologically characteristic, exhibiting as hallmarks of acute GvHD intraepithelial infiltrates of T-lymphocytes and apoptotic target cells; (2) histomorphologically not characteristic, lacking crucial criteria for GvHD and hence not helpful in histological diagnosis; and (3) histomorphologically variable , not caused by GvHD but by microbial infections or drug toxicity, i. e., GvHD-associated lesions. Insufficient awareness of the existence of these three different types of lesions is one of the reasons for the confusion in the literature concerning the histological features of GvHD.

8.1 Histomorphology of GvHD

The present monograph focuses on practical aspects of the clinical and diagnostic pathology of GvHD. It contains abundant illustrations of the gross and microscopic characteristics of GvHD. Appreciation of the clinical appearance is important because diagnosis must be based on clinical as well as pathological findings.

Histologically acute GvHD lesions in the skin, liver, and GIT are characterized by lymphocytic infiltration of the target structures and apoptosis of target cells. No single histopathological phenomenon is specific, pathognomonic for acute GvHD. However, there are histological patterns that are characteristic and in the appropriate clinical context permit the diagnosis of acute GvHD. Such patterns are: lymphocytic interface dermatitis with individual keratinocyte apoptosis, dysplasia and destruction of small bile ducts associated with portal lymphocytic infiltration, increased lymphocytic infiltration of the intestinal mucosa with apoptosis of enterocytes and "exploding crypts." The histological diagnosis of acute GvHD is thus based on pattern analysis, not on the detection of one or two specific morphological phenomena.

In this context it is important to stress that the diagnostic potential of skin, liver, or GIT biopsies in GvHD differs, depending on its purpose. Should the biopsy:

1. Confirm the clinical diagnosis?
2. Establish a diagnosis on its own?
3. Determine the efficacy of GvHD treatment?

Obviously it will be much easier to answer the first and the third question than the second.

The diagnostic reliability of the histological approach can be improved considerably and diagnostic pitfalls can be avoided by optimal timing of biopsies, repeated biopsies, serial sections of tissue probes, and – last but not least – by a close clinicopathological correlation. It should be further understood that whereas the GvHD lesions of the major target organs skin, liver, and GIT are relatively characteristic histologically, GvHD of other organs such as lymph nodes, thymus, and bone marrow shows only cellular depletion and atrophy. Diagnostic pathology therefore concentrates on the three classic target organs of GvHD. This holds true for both acute and chronic GvHD.

8.2 Immunohistology of GvHD

Since histomorphology is frequently insufficient in the recognition of early, mild, or atypical GvHD, the diagnostic potential of immunohistology has been studied intensively. Out of the many immunohistological parameters tested on paraffin sections of GvHD lesions, only the immunophenotypic analysis of inflammatory infiltrates has proved worthwhile diagnostically. CD8$^+$ T-lymphocytes in the epidermis are characteristic of fully developed acute GvHD of the skin. In contrast, OPD4$^+$ T-lymphocytes predominate in the dermis of such lesions. As with histomorphology, no single immunohistological phenomenon is specific or pathognomonic for acute GvHD. That being said, the presence of CD8$^+$ T-lymphocytes in the epidermis, in conjunction with apoptotic keratinocytes, is compatible with the diagnosis of acute GvHD. In contrast, the immunophenotypic analysis of inflammatory infiltrates in the dermis is not discriminatory and is diagnostically irrelevant.

The results of immunophenotyping of inflammatory cells in acute GvHD of the liver and GIT are basically similar to those of the skin. However, the immunohistology of liver and GIT is more difficult to interpret and less informative. Early diagnosis of acute GvHD is possible neither by histomorphology nor by immunohistology. In essence, immunohistological analysis only provides a modest gain of diagnostic information.

8.3 Synopsis of Pathological and Clinical Data on GvHD

The histomorphological evaluation of biopsies in GvHD has diagnostic as well as prognostic relevance. Histological grading of acute and chronic GvHD in the three classic target organs, skin, liver, and GIT, possesses considerable predictive value – in particular if the histological findings are used in conjunction with the clinical data.

Morphological analysis frequently must be done today on biopsies of patients receiving immunosuppressive GvHD prophylaxis or treatment. Under such conditions a reliable histological diagnosis can be very difficult. It is naive to believe that the diagnosis can be based on just one histomorphological, immunohistological, or any other parameter. GvHD diagnosis must be established by a combination of clinical and pathological findings. Clinical and pathological data separately are unreliable. If judiciously combined, a safe diagnosis is possible. As a matter of fact, the clues nowadays to the morphological diagnosis of GvHD are based on a close clinicopathological correlation. Until clinicians find a better means of diagnosis, histomorphology and – to a modest degree – immunohistology will remain useful diagnostic tools in GvHD.

9 Methods Used

Since the present monograph is focused on the clinical and diagnostic pathology of GvHD, the findings presented are exclusively based on the study of formalin-fixed paraffin-embedded tissues, as employed in routine pathology. This applies to the histomorphological and immunohistological investigations performed as well as to the published data cited. This should ensure that the findings reported are relevant to clinical and diagnostic pathology in man.

All biopsies and post mortem tissue probes studied were fixed in 4% buffered formalin for 12–24 h and subsequently embedded in paraffin. For routine histology, immunohistology, and histochemistry, paraffin sections were used throughout. No frozen sections were employed.

9.1 Histological Methods

Routine histological stains and special stains were prepared as described by Romeis [258].

9.2 Immunohistological Methods

Most of the immunohistological studies reported in this monograph were performed retrospectively using paraffin blocks kept in archives. In each instance the tissue specimen was first reexamined histologically for confirmation of the presence of GvHD lesion(s).

Paraffin-embedded biopsies of acute and chronic GvHD of skin, liver, and GIT were studied immunohistologically. Corresponding probes of non-GvHD inflammatory lesions of skin, liver, and GIT served as controls. To unmask antigenic sites paraffin sections were either pretreated with proteases or by microwave exposure. Unfortunately, the latter treatment, although effective in epitope retrieval, frequently resulted in poor structural preservation of tissue sections.

In most of the immunohistological analyses the avidin–biotin complex (ABC)-method was employed [34]. For the detection of $CD3^+$ and $CD8^+$ T-cells the Dako EnVision system was used [36]. To make the immunohistochemical reactions visible, 3-amino-9-ethylcarbazole (AEC) was employed as chromogen. Hematoxylin was used to counterstain the sections.

For immunophenotypic analysis of inflammatory infiltrates, present in GvHD or control lesions, the following panel of primary antibodies (ab) was employed: Polyclonal ab to CD3 (Dako, Code A0452) as a pan T-cell marker, monoclonal ab to CD8 (Dako, Code M7103) as a marker to identify this T-cell subset, monoclonal ab OPD4 (Dako, Code M0834) as a substitute for CD4 specific ab, monoclonal ab to CD57 (BioGenex, Code 314 M) to detect NK1-cells, monoclonal ab to CD20 (Dako, Code M755) as a pan B-cell marker, monoclonal ab to CD68 (Dako, Code M876) to assess cells derived from the monocyte-macrophage lineage, monoclonal ab to CD1a (Immunotech, Code 1590) to identify Langerhans' cells.

ODP4 was employed because CD4 specific antibodies applicable to paraffin sections are not available yet. OPD4 does not selectively recognize $CD4^+$ T-lymphocytes but a larger T-cell subset probably characterized by the CD45RO antigen [89].

For the evaluation of immunohistological reactions a semiquantitative scoring system was used with regard to cells that were labeled: – = none, + = single, ++ = many, and +++ = very numerous (see Fig. 7.4).

9.3 TUNEL Staining

Programmed cell death and simple cell necrosis cannot be distinguished unequivocally by routine histology. Therefore, in situ visualization of apoptosis was achieved by the terminal deoxynucleotidyl transferase (TdT)-mediated dUTP-biotin nick end labeling (TUNEL) method described by Gavrieli et al. [119]. AEC was employed as a chromogen.

References

1. Abbas KA (1995) The immune system: an overview. In: Colvin RB, Bhan AK, McCluskey RT (eds) Diagnostic immunopathology, 2nd edn. Raven, New York, pp 1–22
2. Acevedo A, Aramburu J, Lopez J, Fernandez-Herrera J, Fernandez-Ranada JM, Lopez-Botet M (1991) Identification of natural killer (NK) cells in lesions of human cutaneous graft-versus-host disease: expression of a novel NK-associated surface antigen (Kp43) in mononuclear infiltrates. J Invest Dermatol 97:659–666
3. Ackerman AB (1997) Histologic diagnosis of inflammatory skin diseases. An algorithmic method based on pattern analysis, 2nd edn. Williams and Wilkins, Baltimore
4. Affaticati P, Locatelli F, Roggero S et al (2000) Cytotoxic T lymphocyte precursor frequency as a predictor of acute graft-versus-host disease in bone marrow transplantation from HLA-identical siblings. Bone Marrow Transplant 26:517–523
5. Akpek G, Zahurak ML, Piantadosi S, Margolis J, Doherty J, Davidson R, Vogelsang GB (2001) Development of a prognostic model for grading chronic graft-versus-host disease. Blood 97:1219–1226
6. Alain G, Carrier C, Beaumier L, Bernard J, Lemay M, Lavoie A (1993) In utero acute graft-versus-host disease in a neonate with severe combined immunodeficiency. J Am Acad Dermatol 29:862–865
7. Alam S, Chan KM (1996) Noninfectious pulmonary complications after organ transplantation. Curr –Opin –Pulm Med 2:412–418
8. Anasetti C, Beatty PG, Storb R et al (1990) Effect of HLA incompatibility on graft-versus-host disease, relapse, and survival after marrow transplantation for patients with leukemia or lymphoma. Hum Immunol 29:79–91
9. Andersen CB, Horn T, Sehested M, Junge J, Jacobsen N (1993) Graft-versus-host disease: liver morphology and pheno/genotypes of inflammatory cells and target cells in sex-mismatched allogeneic bone marrow transplant patients. Transplant Proc 25:1250–1254
10. Anderson KC (1997) Transfusion-associated graft-versus-host disease. In: Ferrara JLM, Deeg HJ, Burakoff SJ (1997) Graft-vs-host disease, 2nd edn. Marcel Dekker, New York, pp 587–605
11. Appleton AL, Sviland L (1993) Current thoughts on the pathogenesis of graft-versus-host disease. J Clin Pathol 46:785–789
12. Appleton AL, Sviland L (1994) Immunohistochemistry of transfusion-associated graft-vs.-host disease. Clin Exp Dermatol 19:449–450
13. Appleton AL, Sviland L, Pearson ADJ, Wilkes J, Green MA, Malcolm AJ (1994) Diagnostic features of transfusion associated graft versus host disease. J Clin Pathol 47:541–546
14. Appleton AL, Curtis A, Wilkes J, Cant AJ (1994) Differentiation of materno-fetal GVHD from Omenn's syndrome in pre-BMT patients with severe combined immunodeficiency. Bone Marrow Transplant 14:157–159

15. Aractingi S, Chosidow O (1998) Cutaneous graft-versus-host disease. Arch Dermatol 134:602–612

16. Arai S, Vogelsang GB (2000) Management of graft-versus-host disease. Blood Rev 14:190–204

17. Asplund S, Gramlich TL (1998) Chronic mucosal changes of the colon in graft-versus-host diesease. Mod Pathol 11:513–515

18. Atkinson K (1994) Clinical bone marrow transplantation: a reference textbook. Cambridge University Press, Cambridge

19. Atkinson K (1999) Bone-marrow and blood stem-cell transplantation. In: Berry CL (ed) Transplantation pathology. A guide for practicing pathologists. Springer, Berlin Heidelberg New York, pp 107–136, (Current Topics in Pathology, vol 92)

20. Au WY, Ma SK, Kwong YL et al (2000) Graft-versus-host disease after liver transplantation: documentation by fluorescent in situ hybridisation and human leucocyte antigen typing. Clin Transplant 14:174–177

21. Austin LM, Coven TR, Bhardwaj N, Steinman R, Krueger JG (1998) Intraepidermal lymphocytes in psoriatic lesions are activated GMP-17(TIA-1)+CD8+CD3+ CTLs as determined by phenotypic analysis. J Cutan Pathol 25:79–88

22. Autenrieth IB, Borisch B, Schmeiser T, Arnold R, Jahn G, Müller-Hermelink HK, Heymer B (1989) Stellenwert von Immunhistologie und In-situ-Hybridisierung bei der Differentialdiagnose von Zytomegalievirus-Pneumonie und idiopathischer interstitieller Pneumonie nach allogener Knochenmarktransplantation. Immun Infekt 17:100–108

23. Balduzzi A, Gooley T, Anasetti C et al (1995) Unrelated donor marrow transplantation in children. Blood 86:3247–3256

24. Barksdale SK, Oberlender SA, Barnhill RL (1998) "Rush" skin biopsy specimens in a tertiary medical center: diagnostic yield and clinical utility. J Am Acad Dermatol 38:548–554

25. Baselga E, Drolet BA, Segura AD, Leonardi CL, Esterly NB (1996) Dermatomal lichenoid chronic graft-vs-host disease following varicella-zoster infection despite absence of viral genome. J Cutan Pathol 23:576–581

26. Bauer DJ, Hood AF, Horn TD (1993) Histologic comparison of autologous graft-vs-host reaction and cutaneous eruption of lymphocyte recovery. Arch Dermatol 129:855–858

27. Beelen DW, Elmaagacli A, Müller K-D, Hirche H, Schaefer UW (1999) Influence of intestinal bacterial decontamination using metronidazole and ciprofloxacin or ciprofloxacin alone on the development of acute graft-versus-host disease after marrow transplantation in patients with hematologic malignancies: final results and long-term follow-up of an open-label prospective randomized trial. Blood 93:3267–3275

28. Ben-Ezra JM, Stroup RM (1993) Phenotype of bile ducts and infiltrating lymphocytes in graft-versus-host disease. Transplantation 56:162–165

29. Bensinger WI, Deeg HJ (2000) Blood or marrow? Lancet 355:1199–1200

30. Bensinger WI, Clift RA, Anasetti C, Appelbaum FA, Rowley S, Sandmaier BM, Torok-Storb B (1996) Transplantation of allogeneic peripheral blood stem cells mobilized by recombinant human granulocyte colony stimulating factor. Stem Cells 14:90–105

31. Berry CL (ed) (1999) Transplantation pathology. A guide for practicing pathologists. Springer, Berlin Heidelberg New York, (Current Topics in Pathology, vol 92)

32. Beschorner WE, Farmer ER, Saral R, Stirling WL, Santos GW (1987) Epithelial class II antigen expression in cutaneous graft-versus-host disease. Transplantation 44:237–243
33. Beyer J, Schwerdtfeger R, Siegert W (1992) Graft-versus-host disease or graft-versus-host-like syndrome. Blood 80:2948–2949
34. Bhan AK (1995) Immunoperoxidase. In: Colvin RB, Bhan AK, McCluskey RT (eds) Diagnostic immunopathology, 2nd edn. Raven, New York, pp 711–723
35. Billingham RE (1966–67) The biology of graft-versus-host reactions. Harvey Lect 62:21–78
36. Bisgaard K, Pluzek K (1996) Water soluble polymer conjugates for enzyme immuno assays. 10th International Congress of Histochemistry and Cytochemistry, August 18–23, 1996, Kyoto, Japan. Acta Histochem Cytochem (Suppl) 29:738–739
37. Bligh J, Morton I, Durrant S, Walker N (1995) Oncocytic metaplasia of bile duct epithelium in hepatic GvHD. Bone Marrow Transplant 16:317–319
38. Bochner BS (2000) Road signs guiding leukocytes along the inflammation superhighway. J Allergy Clin Immunol 106:817–828
39. Bombi JA, Palou J, Bruguera M et al (1992) Pathology of bone marrow transplantation. Semin Diagn Pathol 9:220–231
40. Bortin MM, Rimm AA, Saltzstein EC, Rodey GE (1973) Graft versus leukemia. III. Apparent independent antihost and antileukemic activity of transplanted immunocompetent cells. Transplantation 16:182–188
41. Brubaker DB (1986) Transfusion-associated graft-versus-host disease. Hum Pathol 17:1085–1088
42. Buckley RH, Fischer A (1999) Bone marrow transplantation for primary immunodeficiency diseases. In: Ochs HD, Smith CIE, Puck JM (eds) Primary immunodeficiency diseases. A molecular and genetic approach. Oxford University Press, New York, pp 459–475
43. Bunjes D, Theobald M, Nierle T, Arnold R, Heimpel H (1995) Presence of host-specific interleukin 2-secreting T helper cell precursors correlates closely with active primary and secondary chronic graft-versus-host disease. Bone Marrow Transplant 15:727–732
44. Burdick JF, Vogelsang GB, Smith WJ et al (1988) Severe graft-versus-host disease in a liver-transplant recipient. N Engl J Med 318:689–691
45. Burnet M (1969) Self and not-self. Cellular immunology book one. Cambridge University Press, Cambridge
46. Burns LJ, Westberg MW, Burns CP, Klassen LW, Goeken NE, Ray TL, Macfarlane DE (1984) Acute graft-versus-host disease resulting from normal donor blood transfusions. Acta Haematol 71:270–276
47. Byrne JL, Russell NH (1998) Peripheral blood stem cell transplants. J Clin Pathol 51:351–355
48. Cahill RA, Spitzer TR, Mazumder A (1996) Marrow engraftment and clinical manifestations of capillary leak syndrome. Bone Marrow Transplant 18: 177–184
49. Chakrabarti S, Lees A, Jones SG, Milligan DW (2000) Clostridium difficile infection in allogeneic stem cell transplant recipients is associated with severe graft-versus-host disease and non-relapse mortality. Bone Marrow Transplant 26:871–876
50. Chalmers IM, Janossy G, Contreras M, Navarrete C (1998) Intracellular cytokine profile of cord and adult blood lymphocytes. Blood 92:11–18

51. Champlin R (1990) Bone marrow transplantation. Kluwer, Boston
52. Champlin RE, Passweg JR, Zhang M-J et al (2000) T-cell depletion of bone marrow transplants for leukemia from donors other than HLA-identical siblings: advantage of T-cell antibodies with narrow specificities. Blood 95:3996–4003
53. Chao NJ, Deeg HJ (1997) In vivo prevention and treatment of GvHD. In: Ferrara JLM, Deeg HJ, Burakoff SJ (eds) Graft-vs.-host disease, 2nd edn. Marcel Dekker, New York, pp 639–657
54. Chasty RC, Lamb WR, Gallati H, Roberts TE, Brenchley PEC, Yin JAL (1993) Serum cytokine levels in patients undergoing bone marrow transplantation. Bone Marrow Transplant 12:331–336
55. Chaudhuri SPR, Smoller BR (1992) Acute cutaneous graft-versus-host disease: a clinicopathologic and immunophenotypic study. Int J Dermatol 31:270–272
56. Chirletti P, Caronna R, Arcese W, Iori AP, Calcaterra D, Cartoni C, Sammartino P, Stipa V (1998) Gastrointestinal emergencies in patients with acute intestinal graft-versus-host disease. Leuk Lymphoma 29:129–137
57. Clavien PA, Camargo CA Jr, Cameron R, Washington MK, Phillips MJ, Greig PD, Levy GA (1996) Kupffer cell erythrophagocytosis and graft-versus-host hemolysis in liver transplantation. Gastroenterology 110:1891–1896
58. Cohen SB, Perez-Cruz I, Fallen P, Gluckman E, Madrigal JA (1999) Analysis of the cytokine production by cord and adult blood. Hum Immunol 60:331–336
59. Collins RH, Cooper B, Nikaein A, Klintmalm G, Fay JW (1992) Graft-versus-host disease in a liver transplant recipient. Ann Int Med 116:391–392
60. Colvin RB, Bhan AK, McCluskey RT (eds) (1995) Diagnostic immunopathology, 2nd edn. Raven Press, New York
61. Cornelissen JJ (1998) A retrospective Dutch study comparing T cell-depleted allogeneic blood stem cell transplantation vs T cell-depleted allogeneic bone marrow transplantation. Bone Marrow Transplant (Suppl 3) 21:66–70
62. Craven CM, Ward K (1999) Transfusion of fetal cord blood cells: an improved method of hematopoietic stem cell transplantation? J Reprod Immunol 42: 59–77
63. Crawford JM (1997) Graft-versus-host disease of the liver. In: Ferrara JLM, Deeg HJ, Burakoff SJ (eds) Graft-vs.-host disease, 2nd edn. Marcel Dekker, New York, pp 315–336
64. Cruse JM, Lewis RE (1999) Atlas of immunology. CRC Press, Boca Raton; Springer, Berlin Heidelberg New York
65. D'Arena G, Musto P, Cascavilla N, DiGiorgio G, Fusilli S, Zendoli F, Carotenuto M (1998) Flow cytometric characterization of human umbilical cord blood lymphocytes: immunophenotypic features. Haematologica 83:197–203
66. Darmstadt GL, Donnenberg AD, Vogelsang GB, Farmer ER, Horn TD (1992) Clinical, laboratory, and histopathological indicators of the development of progressive acute graft-versus-host disease. J Invest Dermatol 99:397–402
67. Davis RE, Smoller BR (1992) T lymphocytes expressing HECA-452 epitope are present in cutaneous acute graft-versus-host disease and erythema multiforme, but not in acute graft-versus-host disease in gut organs. Am J Pathol 141: 691–698
68. Davison GM, Novitzky N, Kline A, Thomas V, Abrahams L, Hale G, Waldmann H (2000) Immune reconstitution after allogeneic bone marrow transplantation depleted of T cells. Transplantation 69:1341–1347
69. Deeg HJ (1999) Rationale and indications for transplantation. In: Deeg HJ, Klingemann H-G, Phillips GL, van Zant G (eds) A guide to blood and marrow transplantation, 3rd edn. Springer, Berlin Heidelberg New York, pp 7–14

70. Deeg HJ (1999) Graft-versus-host disease (GvHD). In: Deeg HJ, Klingemann H-G, Phillips GL, van Zant G (eds) A guide to blood and marrow transplantation, 3rd edn. Springer, Berlin Heidelberg New York, pp 127–141

71. Deeg HJ (1999) Delayed complications. In: Deeg HJ, Klingemann H-G, Phillips GL, van Zant G (eds) A guide to blood and marrow transplantation, 3rd edn. Springer, Berlin Heidelberg New York, pp 199–203

72. Deeg HJ, Socié G (1998) Malignancies after hematopoietic stem cell transplantation: many questions, some answers. Blood 91:1833–1844

73. Deeg HJ, Storb R (1984) Graft-versus-host disease: pathophysiological and clinical aspects. Ann Rev Med 35:11–24

74. Deeg HJ, Klingemann H-G, Phillips GL, van Zant G (1999) A guide to blood and marrow transplantation, 3rd edn. Springer, Berlin Heidelberg New York

75. Deeg HJ, Flowers MED, Leisenring W, Appelbaum FR, Martin PJ, Storb RF (2000) Cyclosporine (CSP) or CSP plus methylprednisolone for graft-versus-host-disease prophylaxis in patients with high-risk lymphohemopoietic malignancies: long-term follow-up of a randomized trial. Blood 96:1194–1195

76. Demetris AJ (1998) Immune cholangitis: liver allograft rejection and graft-versus-host disease. Mayo Clin Proc 73:367–379

77. DeMeyer ES, Fletcher MA, Buchsel PC (1997) Management of dermatologic complications of chronic graft-versus-host disease: a case study. Clin J Oncol Nurs 1:95–104

78. Demitsu T, Gonda K, Tanita M, Tomita Y (1998) Erythema induced by intra-arterial infusion chemotherapy on the buttock presenting GVHD-like features with marked cellular atypia in histology. Dermatology 197:88–89

79. Desmet VJ (1996) What more can we ask from the pathologist? J Hepatol (Suppl 1) 25:25–29

80. Diamond DJ, Chang KL, Jenkins KA, Forman SJ (1995) Immunohistochemical analysis of T cell phenotypes in patients with graft-versus-host disease following allogeneic bone marrow transplantation. Transplantation 59:1436–1444

81. Dickinson AM, Sviland L, Wang XN, Jackson G, Taylor PR, Dunn A, Proctor SJ (1998) Predicting graft-versus-host disease in HLA-identical bone marrow transplant: a comparison of T-cell frequency analysis and a human skin explant model. Transplantation 66:857–863

82. Donnelly LF, Morris CL (1996) Acute graft-versus-host disease in children: abdominal CT findings. Radiology 199:265–268

83. Drijkoningen M, De Wolf-Peeters C, Tricot G, Degreef H, Desmet V (1988) Drug-induced skin reactions and acute cutaneous graft-versus-host reaction: a comparative immunohistochemical study. Blut 56:69–73

84. Duncker C, Dohr D, von Harsdorf S, Duyster J, Stefanic M, Martini C, Treiber M, Hertenstein B, Novotny J, Arnold R, Heimpel H, Bergmann L, Bunjes D (2000) Non-infectious lung complications are closely associated with chronic graft-versus-host disease: a single center study of incidence, risk factors and outcome. Bone Marrow Transplant 25:1263–1268

85. Dworzak MN, Fröschl G, Printz D, Fleischer C, Pötschger U, Fritsch G, Gadner H, Emminger W (1999) Skin-associated lymphocytes in the peripheral blood of patients with atopic dermatitis: signs of subset expansion and stimulation. J Allergy Clin Immunol 103:901–906

86. Einsele H, Ehninger G, Hebart H et al (1994) Incidence of local CMV infection and acute intestinal GVHD in marrow transplant recipients with severe diarrhoea. Bone Marrow Transplant 14:955–963

87. Einsele H, Waller H-D, Weber P et al (1994) Cytomegalovirus in liver biopsies of marrow transplant recipients: detection methods, clinical, histological and immunohistological features. Med Microbiol Immunol 183:205–216

88. Elliott CJ, Sloane JP, Pallett CD, Sanderson KV (1988) Cutaneous leucocyte composition after human allogeneic bone marrow transplantation: relationship to marrow purging, histology and clinical rash. Histopathology 12:1–16

89. Ellis DW (1993) Lymphoproliferative disorders. In: Leong AS-Y (ed) Applied immunohistochemistry for the surgical pathologist. Edward Arnold, London, pp 110–186

90. Elmaagacli AH, Beelen DW, Trenn G, Schmidt O, Nahler M, Schaefer UW (1999) Induction of a graft-versus-leukemia reaction by cyclosporin A withdrawal as immunotherapy for leukemia relapsing after allogeneic bone marrow transplantation. Bone Marrow Transplant 23:771–777

91. Emile JF, Geissmann F, de la Calle Martin O, Radford-Weiss I, Lepelletier Y, Heymer B, Espanol T, de Santes KB, Bertrand Y, Brousse N, Casanova J-L, Fischer A (2000) Langerhans cell deficiency in reticular dysgenesis. Blood 96:58–62

92. Esteban JM, Somlo G (1995) Skin biopsy in allogeneic and autologous bone marrow transplant patients: a histologic and immunohistochemical study and review of the literature. Mod Pathol 8:59–64

93. Faber LM, van Luxemburg-Heijs SAP, Veenhof WFJ, Willemze R, Falkenburg JHF (1995) Generation of CD4$^+$ cytotoxic T–lymphocyte clones from a patient with severe graft-versus-host disease after allogeneic bone marrow transplantation: implications for graft-versus-leukemia reactivity. Blood 86:2821–2828

94. Farmer ER (2000) Why a skin biopsy? Arch Dermatol 136:779–780

95. Favre A, Cerri A, Bacigalupo A, Lanino E, Berti E, Grossi CE (1997) Immunohistochemical study of skin lesions in acute and chronic graft versus host disease following bone marrow transplantation. Am J Surg Pathol 21:23–34

96. Ferrara JLM (1998) The cytokine modulation of acute graft-versus-host disease, 2nd edn. Bone Marrow Transplant (Suppl 3) 21:S13-S15

97. Ferrara JLM (2000) Cytokines and the regulation of tolerance. J Clin Invest 105:1043–1044

98. Ferrara JLM, Cooke KR, Pan L, Krenger W (1996) The immunopathophysiology of acute graft-versus-host disease. Stem cells 14:473–489

99. Ferrara JLM, Krenger W, Cooke KR et al (1997) Recent advances and future directions. In: Ferrara JLM, Deeg HJ, Burakoff SJ (eds) Graft-vs.-host disease, 2nd edn. Marcel Dekker, New York, pp 775–801

100. Ferrara JLM, Deeg HJ, Burakoff, SJ (1997) Graft-vs.-host disease, 2nd edn. Marcel Dekker, New York

101. Ferrara JLM, Holler E, Blazar B (1999) Monoclonal antibody and receptor antagonist therapy for GVHD. Cancer Treat Res 101:331–368

102. Ferrara JLM, Levy R, Chao NJ (1999) Pathophysiologic mechanisms of acute graft-vs.-host disease. Biol Blood Marrow Transplant 5:347–356

103. Fischer A, Landais P, Friedrich W et al (1990) European experience of bone-marrow transplantation for severe combined immunodeficiency. Lancet 336:850–854

104. Fischer A, Landais P, Friedrich W et al (1994) Bone marrow transplantation (BMT) in Europe for primary immunodeficiencies other than severe combined immunodeficiency: a report from the European group for BMT and the European group for immunodeficiency. Blood 83:1149–1154

105. Fischer A, Haddad E, Jabado N, Casanova JL, Blanche S, Le Deist F, Cavazzana-Calvo M (1998) Stem cell transplantation for immunodeficiency. Springer Semin Immunopathol 19:479–492

106. Fishman JA, Rubin RH (1995) Opportunistic infections. In: Colvin RB, Bhan AK, McCluskey RT (eds) Diagnostic immunopathology, 2nd edn. Raven Press, New York, pp 283–299

107. Flake AW, Zanjani ED (1999) In utero hematopoietic stem cell transplantation: ontogenic opportunities and biologic barriers. Blood 94:2179–2191

108. Foley R, Couban S, Walker I, Greene K, Chen CS, Messner H, Gauldie J (1998) Monitoring soluble interleukin-2 receptor levels in related and unrelated donor allogeneic bone marrow transplantation. Bone Marrow Transplant 21:769–773

109. Forman SJ, Blume KG, Thomas ED (1994) Bone marrow transplantation. Blackwell Scientific Publications, Boston

110. Fowler DH, Gress RE (1997) Graft-versus-host disease as a Th1-type process: regulation by donor cells of Th2 cytokine phenotype. In: Ferrara JLM, Deeg HJ, Burakoff SJ (eds) Graft-vs.-host disease, 2nd edn. Marcel Dekker, New York, pp 479–500

111. Fox H (2000) Is H&E morphology coming to an end? J Clin Pathol 53:38–40

112. Fox RJ, Vogelsang GB, Beschorner WE (1996) Denuded bowel after recovery from graft-versus-host disease. Transplantation 62:1681–1684

113. Friedrich W (1996) Bone marrow transplantation in immunodeficiency diseases. Ann Med 28:115–119

114. Friedrich W, Goldmann SF, Vetter U et al (1984) Immunoreconstitution in severe combined immunodeficiency after transplantation of HLA-haploidentical, T-cell-depleted bone marrow. Lancet 1:761–764

115. Fujii H, Ohashi M, Nagura H (1988) Immunohistochemical analysis of oral lichen-planus-like eruption in graft-versus-host dieesase after allogeneic bone marrow transplantation. Am J Clin Pathol 89:177–186

116. Fujimori Y, Takatsuka H, Takemoto Y, Hara H, Okamura H, Nakanishi K, Kakishita E (2000) Elevated interleukin (IL)-18 levels during acute graft-versus-host disease after allogeneic bone marrow transplantation. Br J Haematol 109:652–657

117. Gale RP, Reisner Y (1986) Graft rejection and graft-versus-host disease: mirror images. Lancet 1:1468–1470

118. Gaschet J, Trevino MA, Cherel M, Vivien R, Garcia-Sahuquillo A, Hallet MM, Bonneville M (1996) HLA-target antigens and T-cell receptor diversity of activated T cells invading the skin during acute graft-versus-host disease. Blood 87: 2345–2353

119. Gavrieli Y, Sherman Y, Ben-Sasson SA (1992) Identification of programmed cell death in situ via specific labeling of nuclear DNA fragmentation. J Cell Biol 119:493–501

120. Gilliam AC, Murphy GF (1997) Cellular pathology of cutaneous graft-versus-host disease. In: Ferrara JLM, Deeg HJ, Burakoff SJ (eds) Graft-vs.-host disease, 2nd edn. Marcel Dekker, New York, pp 291–313

121. Gluckman E, Broxmeyer HA, Auerbach AD et al (1989) Hematopoietic reconstitution in a patient with Fanconi's anemia by means of umbilical-cord blood from an HLA-identical sibling. N Engl J Med 321:1174–1178

122. Gluckman E, Rocha V, Boyer-Chammard A et al (1997) Outcome of cord-blood transplantation from related and unrelated donors. N Engl J Med 337:373–381

123. Glucksberg H, Storb R, Fefer A, Buckner CD, Neiman PE, Clift RA, Lerner KG, Thomas ED (1974) Clinical manifestations of graft-versus-host disease in human recipients of marrow from HL-A-matched sibling donors. Transplantation 18:295–304

124. Gorman TE, Julius CJ, Barth RF et al (2000) Transfusion-associated graft-vs-host disease. A fatal case caused by blood from an unrelated HLA homozygous donor. Am J Clin Pathol 113:732–737

125. Grimm J, Zeller W, Zander AR (1998) Soluble interleukin-2 receptor serum levels after allogeneic bone marrow transplantations as a marker for GvHD. Bone Marrow Transplant 21:29–32

126. Gross TG, Steinbuch M, DeFor T et al (1999) B cell lymphoproliferative disorders following hematopoietic stem cell transplantation: risk factors, treatment and outcome. Bone Marrow Transplant 23:251–258

127. Gruhn B, Hafer R, Kosmehl H, Fuchs D, Zintl F (1998) Cyclosporin A-induced graft-versus-host disease following autologous bone marrow and stem cell transplantation in hematological malignancies of childhood. Bone Marrow Transplant 21:901–907

128. Haddad E, Landais P, Friedrich W et al (1998) Long-term immune reconstitution and outcome after HLA-nonidentical T-cell-depleted bone marrow transplantation for severe combined immunodeficiency: a European retrospective study of 116 patients. Blood 91:3646–3653

129. Hale G, Zhang MJ, Bunjes D et al (1998) Improving the outcome of bone marrow transplantation by using CD52 monoclonal antibodies to prevent graft-versus-host disease and graft rejection. Blood 92:4581–4590

130. Hale G, Jacobs P, Wood L et al (2000) CD52 antibodies for prevention of graft-versus-host disease and graft rejection following transplantation of allogeneic peripheral blood stem cells. Bone Marrow Transplant 26:69–76

131. Handgretinger R, Schumm M, Lang P et al (1999) Transplantation of megadoses of purified haploidentical stem cells. Ann NY Acad Sci 872:351–361

132. Harris DT, Schumacher MJ, LoCascio J, Booth A, Bard J, Boyse EA (1994) Immunoreactivity of umbilical cord blood and post-partum maternal peripheral blood with regard to HLA-haploidentical transplantation. Bone Marrow Transplant 14:63–68

133. Hart DNJ, Fearnley DB (1997) The effect of GvHD on the hematopoietic system. In: Ferrara JLM, Deeg HJ, Burakoff SJ (eds) Graft-vs.-host disease, 2nd edn. Marcel Dekker, New York, pp 447–477

134. Harte G, Payton D, Carmody F, O'Regan P, Thong YH (1997) Graft versus host disease following intrauterine and exchange transfusions for rhesus haemolytic disease. Aust N Z J Obstet Gynaecol 37:319–322

135. Hentschel R, Broecker EB, Kolde G et al (1995) Intact survival with transfusion-associated graft-versus-host disease proved by human leukocyte antigen typing of lymphocytes in skin biopsy specimens. J Pediatr 126:61–64

136. Hepburn NC, McLaren KM, Turner ML, Beveridge GW (1993) The role of skin biopsies in bone marrow transplant recipients. Q J Med 86:715–717

137. Herbay A von, Rudi J (2000) Role of apoptosis in gastric epithelial turnover. Microsc Res Tech 48:303–311

138. Hertenstein B, Wiesneth M, Novotny J et al (1993) Interferon-α and donor buffy coat transfusions for treatment of relapsed chronic myeloid leukemia after allogeneic bone marrow transplantation. Transplantation 56:1114–1118

139. Hervé P, Flesch M, Tiberghien P et al (1992) Phase I-II trial of a monoclonal anti-tumor necrosis factor α antibody for the treatment of refractory severe acute graft-versus-host disease. Blood 79:3362–3368

140. Hess AD (1997) The immunobiology of syngeneic/autologous graft-versus-host disease. In: Ferrara JLM, Deeg HJ, Burakoff SJ (eds) Graft-vs.-host disease, 2nd edn. Marcel Dekker, New York, pp 561–586

141. Heymer B (1985) Causative agents, mediators and histomorphology of inflammation. Pathol Res Pract 180:143–150

142. Heymer B, Krüger G, Arnold R, Schmeiser T, Friedrich W, Kubanek B, Heimpel H (1984) GvH reaction and morphology of bone marrow after allogeneic bone marrow transplantation. In: Lennert K, Hübner K (eds) Pathology of the bone marrow. Gustav Fischer, Stuttgart, pp 281–285

143. Heymer B, Friedrich W, Knobloch C, Goldmann SF (1990) Retikuläre Dysgenesie: Primäre Differenzierungsstörung hämatopoietischer Stammzellen? Verh Dtsch Ges Pathol 74:106–110

144. Heymer B, Hertenstein B, Arnold R, Friedrich W (1993) Problematik der histologischen Diagnostik der Graft-versus-Host-Disease bei Knochenmarktransplantat-Patienten unter GvHD-Prophylaxe. Verh Dtsch Ges Pathol 77:419

145. Heymer B, Friedrich W, Vossbeck S, Negri G, Müller-Hermelink HK (1993) Das sogenannte Omenn-Syndrom. Ein Beitrag zur Pathogenese und Histomorphologie. Pathologe 14:334–340

146. Hill GR, Ferrara JLM (2000) The primacy of the gastrointestinal tract as a target organ of acute graft-versus-host disease: rationale for the use of cytokine shields in allogeneic bone marrow transplantation. Blood 95:2754–2759

147. Hill GR, Krenger W, Ferrara JLM (1997) The role of cytokines in acute graft-versus-host disease. Cytokines Cell Mol Ther 3:257–265

148. Hiroki A, Nakamura S, Shinohara M, Oka M (1994) Significance of oral examination in chronic graft-versus-host disease. J Oral Pathol Med 23:209–215

149. Hitchins L, Fucich LF, Freeman SM, Millikan LE, Marrogi AJ (1997) Immunophenotyping as a diagnostic tool to differentiate lichen planus from chronic graft-versus-host disease: diagnostic observations on two patients. J Invest Med 45:463–468

150. Holler E, Kolb HJ, Möller A et al (1990) Increased serum levels of tumor necrosis factor α precede major complications of bone marrow transplantation. Blood 75:1011–1016

151. Holler E, Kolb HJ, Mittermüller J et al (1995) Modulation of acute graft-versus-host-disease after allogeneic bone marrow transplantation by tumor necrosis factor alpha (TNF alpha) release in the course of pretransplant conditioning: role of conditioning regimens and prophylactic application of a monoclonal antibody neutralizing human TNF alpha (MAK 195F). Blood 86: 890–899

152. Holler E, Kolb HJ, Eissner G, Wilmanns W (1998) Cytokines in GvH and GvL. Bone Marrow Transplant (Suppl 4) 22:S3–6

153. Hood AF, Vogelsang GB, Black LP, Farmer ER, Santos GW (1987) Acute graft-vs-host disease. Development following autologous and syngeneic bone marrow transplantation. Arch Dermatol 123:745–750

154. Horn TD (1994) Acute cutaneous eruptions after marrow ablation: roses by other names? J Cutan Pathol 21:385–392

155. Horn TD (1999) Effector cells in cutaneous graft-versus-host disease. Who? What? When? Where? How? Br J Dermatol 141:779–780

156. Horn TD, Haskell J (1998) The lymphocytic infiltrate in acute cutaneous allogeneic graft-versus-host reactions lacks evidence for phenotypic restriction in donor-derived cells. J Cutan Pathol 25:210–214

157. Horn TD, Lehmkuhle MA, Gore S, Hood A, Burke P (1996) Systemic cytokine administration alters the histology of the eruption of lymphocyte recovery. J Cutan Pathol 23:242–246

158. Horn TD, Zahurak ML, Atkins D, Solomon AR, Vogelsang GB (1997) Lichen planus-like histopathologic characteristics in the cutaneous graft-versus-host reaction. Arch Dermatol 133:961–965

159. Horowitz MM (2000) Current status of allogeneic bone marrow transplantation in acquired aplastic anemia. Semin Hematol 37:30–42

160. Hows JM (2001) Status of umbilical cord blood transplantation in the year 2001. J Clin Pathol 54:428–434

161. Huber J, Zegers BJM, Schuurman H-J (1992) Pathology of congenital immunodeficiencies. Semin Diagn Pathol 9:31–62

162. Hymes SR, Farmer ER, Lewis PG, Tutschka PJ, Santos GW (1985) Cutaneous graft-versus-host reaction: prognostic features seen by light microscopy. J Am Acad Dermatol 12:468–474

163. Imoto S, Oomoto Y, Murata K et al (2000) Kinetics of serum cytokines after allogeneic bone marrow transplantation: interleukin–5 as a potential marker of acute graft-versus-host disease. Int J Hematol 72:92–97

164. Iversen OH (1989) The cell kinetics of the inflammatory reaction. Introduction and overview. In: Iversen OH (ed) Cell kinetics of the inflammatory reaction. Springer, Berlin Heidelberg New York, pp 1–5

165. Jakic-Razumovic J, Browne MD, Sale GE (1992) Proliferation rates in epidermis of patients with graft-versus-host disease, non-specific inflammation and normal skin. Bone Marrow Transplant 10:27–31

166. Jamieson NV, Joysey V, Friend PJ, Marcus R, Ramsbottom S, Baglin T, Johnston PS, Williams R, Calne RY (1991) Graft-versus-host disease in solid organ transplantation. Transplant Int 4:67–71

167. Janossy G, Montano L, Selby WS et al (1982) T cell subset abnormalities in tissue lesions developing during autoimmune disorders, viral infection, and graft-vs.-host disease. J Clin Immunol (Suppl) 2:42S–56 S

168. Jerome KR, Conyers SJ, Hansen DA, Zebala JA (1998) Keratinocyte apoptosis following bone marrow transplantation: evidence for CTL-dependent and -independent pathways. Bone Marrow Transplant 22:359–366

169. Johnson FL, Pochedly C (1990) Bone marrow transplantation in children. Raven, New York

170. Kaserer K, Sedivy R, Mosberger I, Kummer A, Wrba F, Penner E (1996) Charakterisierung des Entzündungszellinfiltrates bei Autoimmun-Cholangitis: Eine immunhistochemische Studie. Verh Dtsch Ges Pathol 80:272–275

171. Kasten-Sportès C, Masset M, Varrin F, Devergie A, Gluckman E (1989) Phenotype and function of T lymphocytes infiltrating the skin during graft-versus-host disease following allogeneic bone marrow transplantation. Transplantion 47:621–624

172. Kaye VN, Neumann PM, Kersey J, Goltz RW, Baldridge BD, Michael AF, Platt JL (1984) Identity of immune cells in graft-versus-host disease of the skin. Analysis using monoclonal antibodies by indirect immunofluorescence. Am J Pathol 116:436–440

173. Klimczak A, Lange A (2000) Apoptosis of keratinocytes is associated with infiltration of CD8$^+$ lymphocytes and accumulation of Ki67 antigen. Bone Marrow Transplant 26:1077–1082

174. Klingebiel T, Schlegel PG (1998) GVHD: overview on pathophysiology, incidence, clinical and biological features. Bone Marrow Transplant (Suppl 2) 21:S45-S49

175. Klingemann H-G (1999) Prevention and treatment of relapse. In: Deeg HJ, Klingemann H-G, Phillips GL, van Zant G (eds) A guide to blood and marrow transplantation, 3rd edn. Springer, Berlin Heidelberg New York, pp 93–97

176. Klingemann H-G (1999) Chronic graft-versus-host disease. In: Deeg HJ, Klingemann H-G, Phillips GL, van Zant G (eds) A guide to blood and marrow transplantation, 3rd edn. Springer, Berlin Heidelberg New York, pp 183–198

177. Klingemann H-G (2000) Relevance and potential of natural killer cells in stem cell transplantation. Biol Blood Marrow Transplant 6:90–99

178. Knutsen AP, Wall DA (1999) Kinetics of T-cell development of umbilical cord blood transplantation in severe T-cell immunodeficiency disorders. J Allergy Clin Immunol 103: 823–832

179. Kobayashi S, Imamura M, Hashino S, Tanaka J, Asaka M (1997) Clinical relevance of serum soluble interleukin-2 receptor levels in acute and chronic graft-versus-host disease. Leuk Lymphoma 28:159–169

180. Kohler S, Hendrickson MR, Chao NJ, Smoller BR (1997) Value of skin biopsies in assessing prognosis and progression of acute graft-versus-host disease. Am J Surg Pathol 21:988–996

181. Kolb HJ, Mittermüller J, Clemm C et al (1990) Donor leukocyte transfusions for treatment of recurrent chronic myelogenous leukemia in marrow transplant patients. Blood 76:2462–2465

182. Kolb HJ, Schattenberg A, Goldman JM et al (1995) Graft-versus-leukemia effect of donor lymphocyte transfusions in marrow grafted patients. Blood 86: 2041–2050

183. Kolbeck PC, Markin RS, McManus BM (1994) Transplant pathology. American Society of Clinical Pathologists, Chicago

184. Kondo M, Kojima S, Horibe K, Kato K, Matsuyama T (2001) Risk factors for chronic graft-versus-host disease after allogeneic stem cell transplantation in children. Bone Marrow Transplant 27:727–730

185. Krampera M, Tavecchia L, Benedetti F, Nadali G, Pizzolo G (2000) Intracellular cytokine profile of cord blood T-, and NK– cells and monocytes. Haematologica 85:675–679

186. Kraus MD, Shahsafaei A, Antin J, Odze RD (1998) Relationship of Bcl-2 expression with apoptosis and proliferation in colonic graft versus host disease. Hum Pathol 29:869–875

187. Kreisel W, Herbst EW, Schwind B, Ochs A, Olschewski M, Köchling G, Fauser AA (1994) Diagnosis and grading of acute graft-versus-host disease following allogeneic bone marrow transplantation by sigmoidoscopy. Eur J Gastroenterol Hepatol 6:723–729

188. Krüger GRF (1985) Klinische Immunpathologie. Kohlhammer-Verlag, Stuttgart, pp 445–453

189. Krüger GRF, Berard CW, DeLellis RA et al (1971) Graft-versus-host disease. Morphologic variation and differential diagnosis in 8 cases of HL-A matched bone marrow transplantation. Am J Pathol 63:179–197

190. Kupper TS (1988) Interleukin 1 and other human keratinocyte cytokines: molecular and functional characterization. Adv Dermatol 3:293–308

191. Kurnick JT, Bhan AK, McCluskey RT (1995) Analysis of cell-mediated reactions. In: Colvin RB, Bhan AK, McCluskey RT (eds) Diagnostic immunopathology, 2nd edn. Raven Press, New York, pp 23–40

192. Kurtzberg J, Laughlin M, Graham ML et al (1996) Placental blood as a source of hematopoietic stem cells for transplantation into unrelated recipients. N Engl J Med 335:157–166

193. Langley RGB, Walsh N, Nevill T, Thomas L, Rowden G (1996) Apoptosis is the mode of keratinocyte death in cutaneous graft-versus-host disease. J Am Acad Dermatol 35:187–190

194. LeBoit PE (1989) Subacute radiation dermatitis: a histologic imitator of acute cutaneous graft-versus-host disease. J Am Acad Dermatol 20:236–241

195. Lee C-K, Gingrich RD, Hohl RJ, Ajram KA (1995) Engraftment syndrome in autologous bone marrow and peripheral stem cell transplantation. Bone Marrow Transplant 16:175–182

196. Lee S, Chong SY, Lee JW, Kim SC, Min YH, Hahn JS, Ko YW (1997) Difference in the expression of Fas/Fas-ligand and the lymphocyte subset reconstitution according to the occurrence of acute GvHD. Bone Marrow Transplant 20:883–888

197. Lerner KG, Kao GF, Storb R, Buckner CD, Clift RA, Thomas ED (1974) Histopathology of graft-vs.-host reaction (GvHR) in human recipients of marrow from HL-A-matched sibling donors. Transplant Proc 6:367–371

198. Leskinen R, Taskinen E, Volin L, Ruutu T, Hayry P (1992) Immunohistology of skin and rectum biopsies in bone marrow transplant recipients. APMIS 100: 1115–1122

199. Liem M, van Lopik T, van Nieuwenhuijze AE, van Houwelingen HC, Aarden L, Goulmy E (1998) Soluble Fas levels in sera of bone marrow transplantation recipients are increased during acute graft-versus-host disease but not during infections. Blood 91:1464–1468

200. Locatelli F, Zecca M, Rondelli R et al (2000) Graft versus host disease prophylaxis with low-dose cyclosporine – A reduces the risk of relapse in children with acute leukemia given HLA-identical sibling bone marrow transplantation: results of a randomized trial. Blood 95:1572–1579

201. MacDonald TT, Spencer J (1992) Cell-mediated immune injury in the intestine. Gastroenterol Clin North Am 21:367–386

202. MacSween RNM, Anthony PP, Scheuer PJ, Burt AD, Portmann BC (1995) Pathology of the liver, 3rd edn. Churchill Livingstone, Edinburgh

203. Madtes DK, Crawford SW (1997) Lung injuries associated with graft-versus-host disease. In: Ferrara JLM, Deeg HJ, Burakoff SJ (eds) Graft-vs.-host disease, 2nd edn. Marcel Dekker, New York, pp 425–446

204. Margolis DA, Casper JT (2000) Alternative-donor hematopoietic stem-cell transplantation for severe aplastic anemia. Semin Hematol 37:43–55

205. Martin P, Nash R, Sanders J, Leisenring W, Anasetti C, Deeg HJ, Storb R, Appelbaum F (1998) Reproducibility in retrospective grading of acute graft-versus-host disease after allogeneic marrow transplantation. Bone Marrow Transplant 21:273–279

206. Martin P, Schoch G, Gooley T, Anasetti C, Deeg HJ, Nash R, Sanders J, Storb R, Appelbaum F (1998) Methods for assessment of graft-versus-host disease. Blood 92:3479–3481

207. Martino R, Romero P, Subira M et al (1999) Comparison of the classic Glucksberg criteria and the IBMTR severity index for grading acute graft-versus-host disease following HLA-identical sibling stem cell transplantation. International Bone Marrow Transplant Registry. Bone Marrow Transplant 24:283–287

208. Massi D, Franchi A, Pimpinelli N, Laszlo D, Bosi A, Santucci M (1999) A reappraisal of the histopathologic criteria for the diagnosis of cutaneous allogeneic acute graft-vs-host disease. Am J Clin Pathol 112:791–800

209. Massumoto C, Benyunes MC, Sale G et al (1996) Close simulation of acute graft-versus-host disease by interleukin-2 administered after autologous bone marrow transplantation for hematologic malignancy. Bone Marrow Transplant 17:351–356

210. McCartan BE, McCreary CE (1997) Oral lichenoid drug eruptions. Oral Dis 3:58–63

211. McDonald GB, Sullivan KM, Schuffler MD, Shulman HM, Thomas ED (1981) Esophageal abnormalities in chronic graft-versus-host disease in humans. Gastroenterology 80:914–921

212. Meyers JD, Thomas ED (1988) Infection complicating bone marrow transplantation. In: Rubin RH, Young LS (eds) Clinical approach to infection in the compromised host. Plenum Medical Book, New York, pp 525–556

213. Miglio F, Pignatelli M, Mazzeo V et al (1987) Expression of major histocompatibility complex class II antigens on bile duct epithelium in patients with hepatic graft-versus-host disease after bone marrow transplantation. J Hepatol 5:182–189

214. Moreb JS, Kubilis PS, Mullins DL, Myers L, Youngblood M, Hutcheson C (1997) Increased frequency of autoaggression syndrome associated with autologous stem cell transplantation in breast cancer patients. Bone Marrow Transplant 19:101–106

215. Morgan G (1992) Bone marrow transplantation for immunodeficiency syndromes. In: Treleaven J, Barrett J (eds) Bone marrow transplantation in practice. Churchill Livingstone, Edinburgh, pp 119–135

216. Mowat A (1997) Intestinal graft-versus-host disease. In: Ferrara JLM, Deeg HJ, Burakoff SJ (eds) Graft-vs.-host disease, 2nd edn. Marcel Dekker, New York, pp 337–384

217. Müller C (1983) Charakterisierung GvH-bedingter Hautläsionen mit Hilfe monoklonaler Antikörper am Gefrierschnitt. Verh Dtsch Ges Pathol 67:362–366

218. Müller SM, Kohn T, Schulz AS, Debatin K-M, Friedrich W (2000) Similar pattern of thymic-dependent T-cell reonstitution in infants with severe combined immunodeficiency after human leukocyte antigen (HLA)-identical and HLA-nonidentical stem cell transplantation. Blood 96:4344–4349

219. Müller-Hermelink HK, Sale GE (1983) Pathologische Befunde bei Knochenmarkstransplantation. Verh Dtsch Ges Pathol 67:335–361

220. Müller-Ruchholtz W (1990) The immunopathology of transplantation. In: Sale GE (ed) The pathology of organ transplantation. Butterworths, Boston, pp 1–24

221. Myerowitz RL (1983) The pathology of opportunistic infections. With pathogenetic, diagnostic, and clinical correlations. Raven Press, New York

222. Naeim F (1992) Pathology of bone marrow. Igaku-Shoin, New York

223. Naeim F, Gale RP (1992) Bone marrow transplantation. In: Naeim F (ed) Pathology of bone marrow. Igaku-Shoin, New York, pp 343–355

224. Nagler RM, Sherman Y, Nagler A (1999) Histopathological study of the human submandibular gland in graft versus host disease. J Clin Pathol 52:395–397

225. Nelson JL, Furst DE, Maloney S et al (1998) Microchimerism and HLA-compatible relationships of pregnancy in scleroderma. Lancet 351:559–562

226. Neumann UP, Kaisers U, Langrehr JM et al (1994) Fatal graft-versus-host disease: a grave complication after orthotopic liver transplantation. Transplant Proc 26:3616–3617

227. Nghiem P (2001) The "drug vs graft-vs-host disease" conundrum gets tougher, but there is an answer. The challenge to dermatologists. Arch Dermatol 137: 75–76

228. Niederwieser D, Herold M, Woloszczuk W et al (1990) Endogenous IFN-gamma during human bone marrow transplantation. Analysis of serum levels of interferon and interferon-dependent secondary messages. Transplantation 50:620–625

229. Niederwieser D, Grassegger A, Auböck J et al (1993) Correlation of minor histocompatibility antigen-specific cytotoxic T lymphocytes with graft-versus-host disease status and analyses of tissue distribution of their target antigens. Blood 81:2200–2208

230. Nierhoff D, Horvath HC, Mytilineos J et al (2000) Microchimerism in bone marrow-derived CD34$^+$ cells of patients after liver transplantation. Blood 96:763–767

231. Nierle T, Bunjes D, Arnold R, Heimpel H, Theobald M (1993) Quantitative assessment of posttransplant host-specific interleukin – 2-secreting T-helper cell precursors in patients with and without acute graft-versus-host disease after allogeneic HLA-identical sibling bone marrow transplantation. Blood 81: 841–848

232. Niethammer D, Goldmann SF, Flad H-D et al (1979) Graft-versus-host reaction after blood transfusion in a patient with cellular immunodeficiency: the role of histocompatibility testing. Eur J Pediatr 132:43–48

233. Noga SJ, Civin CI (1997) Positive stem-cell selection for hematopoetic transplantation. In: Ferrara JLM, Deeg HJ, Burakoff SJ(eds) Graft-vs.-host disease, 2nd edn. Marcel Dekker, New York, pp 717–731

234. Norton J, Sloane JP (1992) Epidermal damage in skin of allogeneic marrow recipients: relative importance of chemotherapy, conditioning and graft v. host disease. Histopathology 21:529–534

235. Norton J, Sloane JP (1994) A prospective study of cellular immunologic changes in skin of allogeneic bone marrow recipients. Am J Clin Pathol 101:597–602

236. Nuckols JD, Shea CR, Horenstein MG, Burchette JL, Prieto VG (1999) Quantitation of intraepidermal T-cell subsets in formalin-fixed, paraffin-embedded tissue helps in the diagnosis of mycosis fungoides. J Cutan Pathol 26:169–175

237. Orlin JB, Ellis MH (1997) Transfusion-associated graft-versus-host disease. Curr Opin Hematol 4:442–448

238. Osawa J, Kitamura K, Saito S, Ikezawa Z, Nakajima H (1994) Immunohistochemical study of graft-versus-host reaction (GvHR) – type drug eruptions. J Dermatol 21:25–30

239. Pablos JL, Santiago B, Galindo M, Carreira PE, Ballestin C, Gomez-Reino JJ (1999) Keratinocyte apoptosis and p53 expression in cutaneous lupus and dermatomyositis. J Pathol 188:63–68

240. Palmas A, Tefferi A, Myers JL et al (1998) Late-onset noninfectious pulmonary complications after allogeneic bone marrow transplantation. Br J Haematol 100:680–687

241. Parker P, Chao NJ, Ben-Ezra J et al (1996) Polymyositis as a manifestation of chronic graft-versus-host disease. Medicine 75:279–285

242. Parkman R (1998) Chronic graft-versus-host disease. Curr Opin Hematol 5: 22–25

243. Parrish RS, Hazlett LJ, Bridges KD, Henslee-Downey PJ (1999) A multivariate approach for assessing severity of acute graft-versus-host disease in bone marrow transplantation. Stat Med 18:423–440

244. Perez-Atayde AR, Rosen FS (1995) Pathology of the primary immunodeficiency diseases. In: Colvin RB, Bhan AK, McCluskey RT (eds) Diagostic immunopathology, 2nd edn. Raven Press, New York, pp 241–259

245. Peters C, Minkov M, Gadner H et al (2000) Statement of current majority practices in graft-versus-host disease prophylaxis and treatment in children. Bone Marrow Transplant 26:405–411

246. Pflieger H (1983) Graft-versus-host disease following blood transfusions. Blut 46:61–66

247. Ponec RJ, Hackman RC, McDonald GB (1999) Endoscopic and histologic diagnosis of intestinal graft-versus-host disease after marrow transplantation. Gastrointest Endosc 49:612–621

248. Porta F, Friedrich W (1998) Bone marrow transplantation in congenital immunodeficiency diseases. Bone Marrow Transplant (Suppl 2) 21:S21–S23

249. Portmann B, Koukoulis G (1999) Pathology of the liver allograft. In: Berry CL (ed) Transplantation pathology. A guide for practicing pathologists. Springer, Berlin Heidelberg New York, pp 62–85 (Current Topics in Pathology, vol 92)

250. Powles R, Mehta J, Kulkarni S et al (2000) Allogeneic blood and bone-marrow stem-cell transplantation in haematological malignant diseases: a randomised trial. Lancet 355:1231–1237

251. Przepiorka D, Weisdorf D, Martin P, Klingemann HG, Beatty P, Hows J, Thomas ED (1995) Meeting report. Consensus conference on acute GvHD grading. Bone Marrow Transplant 15:825–828

252. Puck JM (1999) X-linked severe combined immunodeficiency. In: Ochs HD, Smith CIE, Puck JM (eds) Primary immunodeficiency diseases. A molecular and genetic approach. Oxford University Press, New York, pp 99–110

253. Quaranta S, Shulman H, Ahmed A et al (1999) Autoantibodies in human chronic graft-versus-host disease after hematopoietic cell transplantation. Clin Immunol 91:106–116

254. Rhoades JL, Cibull ML, Thompson JS et al (1993) Role of natural killer cells in the pathogenesis of human acute graft-versus-host disease. Transplantation 56:113–120

255. Ringdén O, Deeg HJ (1997) Clinical spectrum of graft-versus-host disease. In: Ferrara JLM, Deeg HJ, Burakoff SJ (eds) Graft-vs.-host disease. Marcel Dekker, New York, pp 525–559

256. Robert C, Kupper TS (1999) Inflammatory skin diseases, T cells, and immune surveillance. N Engl J Med 341:1817–1828

257. Roberts JP, Ascher NL, Lake J, Capper J, Purohit S, Garovoy M, Lynch R, Ferrell L, Wright T (1991) Graft vs. host disease after liver transplantation in humans: a report of four cases. Hepatology 14:274–281

258. Romeis B (1989) Mikroskopische Technik. Neubearbeitung: Böck P (Hrsg) Romeis – Mikroskopische Technik, 17. Aufl. Urban und Schwarzenberg, München, S 235–249

259. Rowbottom AW, Riches PG, Downie C, Hobbs JR (1993) Monitoring cytokine production in peripheral blood during acute graft-versus-host disease following allogeneic bone marrow transplantation. Bone Marrow Transplant 12:635–641

260. Rowlings PA, Przepiorka D, Klein JP et al (1997) IBMTR severity index for grading acute graft-versus-host disease: retrospective comparison with Glucksberg grade. Br J Haematol 97:855–864

261. Roy J, Snover D, Weisdorf S, Mulvahill A, Filipovich A, Weisdorf D (1991) Simultaneous upper and lower endoscopic biopsy in the diagnosis of intestinal graft-versus-host disease. Transplantation 51:642–646

262. Rubeiz N, Taher A, Salem Z, Gharzuddine W, Kibbi AG (1993) Posttransfusion graft-versus-host disease in two immunocompetent patients. J Am Acad Dermatol 28:862–865

263. Rubinstein P, Carrier C, Scaradavou A et al (1998) Outcomes among 562 recipients of placental-blood transplants from unrelated donors. N Engl J Med 339:1565–1577

264. Rubinstein P, Adamson JW, Stevens C (1999) The Placental/Umbilical Cord Blood Program of the New York Blood Center. A progress report. Ann NY Acad Sci 872:328–334

265. Sale GE (1984) Pathology of the lymphoreticular system. In: Sale GE, Shulman HM (eds) The pathology of bone marrow transplantation. Masson, New York, pp 171–191

266. Sale GE (1984) Pathology of bone marrow with marrow transplantation. In: Sale GE, Shulman HM (eds) The pathology of bone marrow transplantation. Masson, New York, pp 215–230

267. Sale GE (1990) The pathology of organ transplantation. Butterworths, Boston

268. Sale GE (1990) Bone marrow and thymic transplantation. In: Sale GE (ed) The pathology of organ transplantation. Butterworths, Boston, pp 229–259

269. Sale GE (1996) Does graft-versus-host disease attack epithelial stem cells? Mol Med Today 2:114–119

270. Sale GE, Hackman RC (1984) Pathology of infections after bone marrow transplantation. In: Sale GE, Shulman HM (eds) The pathology of bone marrow transplantation. Masson, New York, pp 199–214

271. Sale GE, Shulman HM (1984) The pathology of bone marrow transplantation. Masson, New York

272. Sale GE, Lerner KG, Barker EA, Shulman HM, Thomas ED (1977) The skin biopsy in the diagnosis of acute graft-versus-host disease in man. Am J Pathol 89:621–636

273. Sale GE, Shulman HM, McDonald GB, Thomas ED (1979) Gastrointestinal graft-versus-host disease in man. A clinicopathologic study of the rectal biopsy. Am J Surg Pathol 3:291–299

274. Sale GE, Anderson P, Browne M, Myerson D (1992) Evidence of cytotoxic T-cell destruction of epidermal cells in human graft-vs-host disease. Immunohistology with monoclonal antibody TIA-1. Arch Pathol Lab Med 116: 622–625

275. Sale GE, Beauchamp MD, Akiyama M (1994) Parafollicular bulges, but not hair bulb keratinocytes, are attacked in graft-versus-host disease of human skin. Bone Marrow Transplant 14:411–413

276. Sale GE, Beauchamp M, Myerson D (1994) Immunohistologic staining of cytotoxic T and NK cells in formalin-fixed paraffin-embedded tissue using microwave TIA-1 antigen retrieval. Transplantion 57:287–289

277. Sale GE, Shulman HM, Hackman RC (1995) Bone marrow. In: Colvin RB, Bhan AK, McCluskey (eds) Diagnostic immunopathology, 2nd edn. Raven Press, New York, pp 435–453

278. Sale GE, Shulman HM, Hackman RC (1999) Pathology of hematopoietic cell transplantation. In: Thomas ED, Blume KG, Forman SJ (eds) Hematopoietic cell transplantation, 2nd edn. Blackwell Science Inc, Malden, pp 248–263

279. Sanders JE (1990) Late effects following marrow transplantation. In: Johnson FL, Pochedly C (eds) Bone marrow transplantation in children. Raven, New York, pp 471–496

280. Schwarz K, Notarangelo LD, Spanopoulou E, Vezzoni P, Villa A (1999) Recombination defects. In: Ochs HD, Smith CIE, Puck JM (eds) Primary immunodeficiency diseases. A molecular and genetic approach. Oxford University Press, New York, pp 155–166

281. Seemayer TA (1979) The graft-versus-host reaction: a pathogenetic mechanism of experimental and human disease. Perspect Pediatr Pathol 5:93–136

282. Shenoy S, Mohanakumar T, Todd G et al (1999) Immune reconstitution following allogeneic peripheral blood stem cell transplants. Bone Marrow Transplant 23:335–346

283. Sherer Y, Shoenfeld Y (1998) Autoimmune diseases and autoimmunity post-bone marrow transplantation. Bone Marrow Transplant 22:873–881

284. Shulman HM, Sale GE, Lerner KG et al (1978) Chronic cutaneous graft-versus-host disease in man. Am J Pathol 91:545–570

285. Shulman HM, Sullivan KM, Weiden PL et al (1980) Chronic graft-versus-host syndrome in man. A long-term clinicopathologic study of 20 Seattle patients. Am J Med 69:204–217

286. Shulman HM, Sharma P, Amos D, Fenster LF, McDonald GB (1988) A coded histologic study of hepatic graft-versus-host disease after human bone marrow transplantation. Hepatology 8:463–470

287. Siegert W, Stemerowicz R, Hopf U (1992) Antimitochondrial antibodies in patients with chronic graft-versus-host disease. Bone Marrow Transplant 10:221–227

288. Slavin RE, Santos GW (1973) The graft versus host reaction in man after bone marrow transplantation: pathology, pathogenesis, clinical features, and implication. Clin Immunol Immunopathol 1:472–498

289. Slavin RE, Woodruff JM (1974) The pathology of bone marrow transplantation. Pathol Annu 9:291–344

290. Slavin S (1984) Bone marrow and organ transplantation. Elsevier, Amsterdam

291. Sloane JP, Norton J (1993) The pathology of bone marrow transplantation. Histopathology 22:201–209

292. Sloane JP, Depledge MH, Powles RL, Morgenstern GR, Trickey BS, Dady PJ (1983) Histopathology of the lung after bone marrow transplantation. J Clin Pathol 36:546–554

293. Snover DC (1990) Graft-versus-host disease of the gastrointestinal tract. Am J Surg Pathol (Suppl 1) 14:101–108

294. Snover DC, Weisdorf SA, Vercellotti GM, Rank B, Hutton S, McGlave P (1985) A histopathologic study of gastric and small intestinal graft-versus-host disease following allogeneic bone marrow transplantation. Hum Pathol 16:387–392

295. Snover DC, Filipovich AH, Ramsay NKC, Weisdorf SA, Kersey JH (1985) Graft-versus-host-disease-like histopathological findings in pre-bone-marrow transplantation biopsies of patients with severe T cell deficiency. Transplantation 39:95–97

296. Socie G, Stone JV, Wingard JR, Weisdorf D, Henslee-Downey PJ, Bredeson C, Cahn JY, Passweg JR, Rowlings PA, Schouten HC, Kolb HJ, Klein JP (1999) Long-term survival and late deaths after allogeneic bone marrow transplantation. Late Effects Working Committee of the International Bone Marrow Transplant Registry. N Engl J Med 341:14–21

297. Sosman J, Hong R, Sondel PM (1990) Etiology and pathogenesis of graft-vs.-host disease. II. Human studies. In: Johnson FL, Pochedly C (eds) Bone marrow transplantation in children. Raven Press, New York, pp 365–379

298. Spencer GD, Shulman HM, Myerson D, Thomas ED, McDonald GB (1986) Diffuse intestinal ulceration after marrow transplantation: a clinicopathologic study of 13 patients. Hum Pathol 17:621–633

299. Spitzer TR, Cahill R, Cottler-Fox M, Treat J, Sacher R, Deeg HJ (1990) Transfusion-induced graft-versus-host disease in patients with malignant lymphoma. A case report and review of the literature. Cancer 66:2346–2349

300. Springmeyer SC, Silvestri RC, Flournoy N, Kosanke CW, Peterson DL, Huseby JS, Hudson LD, Storb R, Thomas ED (1984) Pulmonary function of marrow transplant patients. I. Effects of marrow infusion, acute graft-versus-host disease, and interstitial pneumonitis. Exp Hematol 12:805–810

301. Stephan JL, Vlekova V, Le Deist F et al (1993) Severe combined immunodeficiency: a retrospective single-center study of clinical presentation and outcome in 117 patients. J Pediatr 123:564–572

302. Storb R, Leisenring W, Anasetti C et al (1997) Methotrexate and cyclosporine for graft-vs.-host disease prevention: what length of therapy with cyclosporine? Biol Blood Marrow Transplant 3:194–201

303. Storb R, Yu C, Sandmaier BM, McSweeney PA, Georges G, Nash RA, Woolfrey A (1999) Mixed hematopoietic chimerism after marrow allografts. Transplantation in the ambulatory care setting. Ann NY Acad Sci 872:372–376

304. Storek J, Gooley T, Siadak M et al (1997) Allogeneic peripheral blood stem cell transplantation may be associated with a high risk of chronic graft-versus-host disease. Blood 90:4705–4709

305. Sullivan KM (1986) Acute and chronic graft-versus-host disease in man. Int J Cell Cloning (Suppl 1) 4:42–93

306. Sullivan KM (1999) Graft-versus-host disease. In: Thomas ED, Blume KG, Forman SJ (eds) Hematopoietic cell transplantation, 2nd edn. Blackwell Science Inc, Malden, pp 515–536

307. Sullivan KM, Deeg HJ, Sanders J et al (1986) Hyperacute graft-v-host disease in patients not given immunosuppression after allogeneic marrow transplantation. Blood 67:1172–1175

308. Sviland L, Dickinson AM (1999) A human skin explant model for predicting graft-versus-host disease following bone marrow transplantation. J Clin Pathol 52:910–913

309. Sviland L, Pearson ADJ, Green MA et al. (1989) Expression of MHC class I and II antigens by keratinocytes and enterocytes in acute graft-versus-host disease. Bone Marrow Transplant 4:233–238

310. Sviland L, Pearson ADJ, Green MA, Eastham EJ, Hamilton PJ, Proctor SJ, Malcolm AJ (1993) Prognostic importance of histological and immunopathological assessment of skin and rectal biopsies in patients with GvHD. Bone Marrow Transplant 11:215–218

311. Sviland L, Pearson ADJ, Hamilton PJ (1994) Diagnosis of acute graft-versus host disease using skin and rectal biopsies. In: Kolbeck PC, Markin RS, McManus BM (eds) Transplant pathology. American Society of Clinical Pathologists, Chicago, pp 293–307

312. Symington FW, Sullivan Pepe M, Chen AB, Deliganis A (1990) Serum tumor necrosis factor alpha associated with acute graft-versus-host disease in humans. Transplantation 50:518–521

313. Takata M, Imai T, Hirone T (1993) Immunoelectron microscopy of acute graft versus host disease of the skin after allogeneic bone marrow transplantation. J Clin Pathol 46:801–805

314. Tanaka M, Umihara J, Shimmoto K, Cui S, Sata H, Ishikawa T, Ishikawa E (1989) The pathogenesis of graft-versus-host reaction in the intrahepatic bile duct. An immunohistochemical study. Acta Pathol Jpn 39:648–655

315. Tanaka Y, Kami M, Ogawa S et al (2000) Hyperacute graft-versus-host disease and NKT cells. Am J Hematol 63:60–61

316. Tanei R, Ohta Y, Ishihara S, Katsuoka K, Yokono H, Motoori T (1999) Transfusion-associated graft-versus-host disease: an in situ hybridization analysis of the infiltrating donor-derived cells in the cutaneous lesion. Dermatology 199: 20–24

317. Theobald M, Nierle T, Bunjes D, Arnold R, Heimpel H (1992) Host-specific interleukin-2-secreting donor T-cell precursors as predictors of acute graft-versus-host disease in bone marrow transplantation between HLA-identical siblings. N Engl J Med 327:1613–1617

318. Theobald M, Nierle T, Bunjes D, Arnold R, Heimpel H (1993) Quantitative assessment of posttransplant host-specific interleukin–2-secreting T–helper cell precursors in patients with and without acute graft-versus-host disease after allogeneic HLA-identical sibling bone marrow transplantation. Blood 81:841–848

319. Thomas ED (1983) Bone marrow transplantation. A lifesaving applied art. JAMA 249:2528–2536

320. Thomas ED (1997) Foreword. In: Ferrara ILM, Deeg HJ, Burakoff SJ (eds) Graft-vs.-host disease, 2nd edn. Marcel Dekker, New York, pp III-IV

321. Thomas ED, Storb R, Clift RA et al (1975) Bone-marrow transplantation. N Engl J Med 292:895–902

322. Thomas ED, Clift RA, Storb R (1984) Indications for marrow transplantation. Ann Rev Med 35:1–9

323. Thomas ED, Blume KG, Forman SJ (1999) Hematopoietic cell transplantation, 2nd edn. Blackwell Science, Inc, Malden

324. Thomson BG, Robertson KA, Gowan D et al (2000) Analysis of engraftment, graft-versus-host disease, and immune recovery following unrelated donor cord blood transplantation. Blood 96:2703–2711

325. Treleaven J, Barrett J (1992) Bone marrow transplantation in practice. Churchill Livingstone, Edinburgh

326. Tzung SP Hackman RC, Hockenbery DM, Bensinger W, Schiffman K, McDonald GB (1998) Lymphocytic gastritis resembling graft-vs.-host disease following autologous hematopoietic cell transplantation. Biol Blood Marrow Transplant 4:43–48

327. Valks R, Fernández-Herrera J, Bartolomé B, Fraga J, Daudén E, Garcia-Diéz A (2001) Late appearance of acute graft-vs-host disease after suspending or tapering immunosuppressive drugs. Arch Dermatol 137:61–65

328. van Dijk AM, Otten HG, Kessler FL, de Boer M, de Gast GC (1997) Detection of keratinocyte-specific helper T-lymphocyte precursor cells for prediction of acute graft-versus-host disease. Transplant Proc 29:720–721

329. Vega RA (1990) Graft-vs.-host disease: hepatic, gastrointestinal, and dermal toxicities. In: Johnson FL, Pochedly C (eds) Bone marrow transplantation in children. Raven Press, New York, pp 381–396

330. Vermeer BJ, van der Spek-Keijser LMT, Fibbe WE (1994) Skin biopsies in bone marrow transplantation. Lancet 344:75–76

331. Vogelsang GB (1990) Transfusion-associated graft-versus-host disease in non-immunocompromised hosts. Transfusion 30:101–103

332. Vogelsang GB (2001) How I treat chronic graft-versus-host disease. Blood 97:1196–1201

333. Vogelsang GB, Hess AD (1994) Graft-versus-host disease: new directions for a persistent problem. Blood 84:2061–2067

334. Volc-Platzer B (1992) „Graft-versus-host disease" (GvHD). Hautarzt 43:669–677

335. Wagner IL, Flowers MED, Longton G, Storb R, Schubert M, Sullivan KM (1998) The development of chronic graft-versus-host disease: an analysis of screening studies and the impact of corticosteroid use at 100 days after transplantation. Bone Marrow Transplant 22:139–146

336. Wakabayashi T, Onoda H, Masunaga A and the Bone Marrow Transplantation Group (1999) Fas/Apo–1 expression of human GVHD livers. Transplant Proc 31:423–424

337. Walker MW, Lovell MA, Kelly TE, Golden W, Saulsbury FT (1993) Multiple areas of intestinal atresia associated with immunodeficiency and posttransfusion graft-versus-host disease. J Pediatr 123:93–95

338. Washington K, Stenzel TT, Buckley RH, Gottfried MR (1996) Gastrointestinal pathology in patients with common variable immunodeficiency and X-linked agammaglobulinemia. Am J Surg Pathol 20:1240–1252

339. Washington K, Bentley RC, Green A, Olson J, Treem WR, Krigman HR (1997) Gastric graft-versus-host disease: a blinded histologic study. Am J Surg Pathol 21:1037–1046

340. Weber-Nordt RM, Schott E, Finke J, Henschler R, Schulz G, Mertelsmann R (1996) Umbilical cord blood: an alternative to the transplantation of bone marrow stem cells. Cancer Treat Rev 22:381–391

341. Weyers W, Bonczkowitz M, Weyers I (1996) Differentialdiagnose der Interface-Dermatitis. Verh Dtsch Ges Pathol 80:241–246

342. Whitehead R (1995) Gastrointestinal and oesophageal pathology, 2nd edn. Churchill Livingstone, Edinburgh

343. Wickenhauser C, Thiele J (1995) Zytokine und Hämatopoese. Pathologe 16:181–191

344. Wickenhauser C, Thiele J, Kümmel T, Fischer R (1995) Die hämatopoietische Stammzelle des Menschen. Pathologe 16:1–10

345. Wisecarver JL, Cattral MS, Langnas AN, Shaw BW, Fox IJ, Heffron TG, Rubocki RJ (1994) Transfusion-induced graft-versus-host disease after liver transplantation. Transplantation 58:269–271

346. Witherspoon RP, Lum LG, Storb R (1984) Immunologic reconstitution after human marrow grafting. Semin Hematol 21:2–10

347. Woodruff JM, Hansen JA, Good RA, Santos GW, Slavin RE (1976) The pathology of the graft-versus-host reaction (GvHR) in adults receiving bone marrow transplants. Transplant Proc 8:675–684

348. Wu D, Hockenberry DM, Brentnall TA et al (1998) Persistent nausea and anorexia after marrow transplantation: a prospective study of 78 patients. Transplantation 66:1319–1324

349. Yamada H, Chihara J, Hamada K, Matsukura M, Yudate T, Maeda K, Tubaki K, Tezuka T (1997) Immunohistology of skin and oral biopsies in graft-versus-host disease after bone marrow transplantation and cytokine therapy. J Allergy Clin Immunol 100:S73-S76

350. Yanik G, Levine JE, Ratanatharathorn V, Dunn R, Ferrara J, Hutchinson RJ (2000) Tacrolimus (FK506) and methotrexate as prophylaxis for acute graft-versus-host disease in pediatric allogeneic stem cell transplantation. Bone Marrow Transplant 26:161–167

351. Yousem SA (1995) The histological spectrum of pulmonary graft-versus-host disease in bone marrow transplant recipients. Hum Pathol 26:668–675

352. Zhou Y, Barnett MJ, Rivers JK (2000) Clinical significance of skin biopsies in the diagnosis and management of graft-vs-host disease in early postallogeneic bone marrow transplantation. Arch Dermatol 136:717–721

Subject Index